The Menopause Solution

Navigating Hormonal Changes
With Hormone Replacement
Therapy, Natural Remedies,
Supplements, and a Healthy
Lifestyle

Stella Sparks

of the information contained within this document, including, but not limited to, errors, omissions, or inaccuracies.

Table of Contents

INTRODUCTION 1

CHAPTER 1: AN OVERVIEW OF MENOPAUSE 5

MENOPAUSE EXPLAINED 5
  The Three Stages of Menopause 6
  Other Possibilities 8
SIGNS AND SYMPTOMS OF MENOPAUSE 8
  Hot Flashes 9
  Changes in Mood 12
  Memory Issues 13
  Anxiety and Depression 14
  Sleep Troubles 15
  Changed Attitude Toward Sex 17
  Irregular Bleeding and Periods 18
  Vaginal Complications 19
  Urinary Issues 20
TO SUMMARIZE 21

CHAPTER 2: HORMONAL CHANGES DURING MENOPAUSE ... 23

THE CAUSE OF MENOPAUSE 23
  Estrogen 24
  Progesterone 24
TREATING MENOPAUSE 25
MEDICINES FOR MENOPAUSE 26
  Hormone Therapy 26
  Selective Estrogen Receptor Modulators 28
  Strontium Ranelate 28
  Bisphosphonates 29
  Low-Dose Hormonal Birth Control 30
  Bioidentical Hormone Therapy 30
  Antidepressants 31

Pregabalin and Gabapentin...33
Topical Vaginal Estrogen 34
Over-the-Counter Products..37
To Summarize 37

CHAPTER 3: HORMONE REPLACEMENT THERAPY 39

An Overview of Hormone Replacement Therapy.....................39
Risks and Benefits of Hormone Replacement Therapy 40
Risks and Considerations of Hormone Replacement
Therapy..41
Benefits of Hormone Replacement Therapy....................42
Controversy Surrounding Hormone Replacement Therapy 44
Hormone Replacement Therapy and Breast Cancer Risk 44
Cardiovascular Effects of Hormone Therapy 45
Alternatives to Hormone Therapy 45
Long-Term Effects of Early Menopause...........................45
Individualized Approaches and Shared Decision-Making 46
Guidelines for Using Hormone Replacement Therapy 47
Individualized Approach 47
Symptom Severity and Impact...47
Timing of Initiation 48
Shortest Duration and Lowest Effective Dose.................48
Combination or Estrogen-Only Therapy 48
Regular Reassessment...48
Individual Health Risks and Considerations....................49
To Summarize 49

CHAPTER 4: SUPPLEMENTS FOR MENOPAUSE 51

Do Supplements Work? 51
Supplements for Managing Menopause Symptoms.................52
Calcium..53
Vitamin D...54
Vitamin E 55
Vitamin C 56
B Vitamins 56
Vitamin A...58
Iron 58
Fluoride..59

To Summarize 60

CHAPTER 5: NATURAL REMEDIES FOR MENOPAUSE 63

Herbal Supplements 64
    Ground Flaxseed 64
    Black Cohosh 65
    Red Clover 67
    Soy 68
    Evening Primrose Oil 69
    Maca 70
    Ginseng 71
    Chasteberry 72
    Valerian 73
    Dong Quai 74
    Wild Yam 75
Flaxseed Oil and Vitamin E 75
To Summarize 76

CHAPTER 6: MENTAL HEALTH AND MENOPAUSE 77

The Impact of Menopause on Mental Health 77
    Contributing Factors 79
Treating Menopause-Related Mental Health Issues 81
    Therapy 81
    Medications 84
    Aromatherapy Massage 85
Dealing With Menopause-Related Mental Health Issues 86
    Prioritize Self-Care 86
    Make Lifestyle Changes 86
To Summarize 87

CHAPTER 7: BENEFICIAL LIFESTYLE CHANGES 89

Eat Foods Rich in Phytoestrogen, Calcium, and Iron 90
    Phytoestrogen-Rich Foods 90
    Calcium-Rich Foods and Vitamin D 93
    Iron-Rich Foods 96
Avoid Trigger Foods 97
Eat Plenty of Fruits and Vegetables 98
Eat Protein-Rich Foods 99

Eat Less Processed Food and Refined Sugar 99

Don't Skip Meals 100

Stay Hydrated 100

Manage Your Weight 101

    Vegetarian/Vegan Diet.. 102

    Mediterranean Diet... 104

    Low Carb Diet 105

Exercise Regularly.. 107

    Strength Training... 108

    Cardio 108

    Dancing... 111

    Yoga.. 112

    Tai Chi... 112

    Pilates 113

    Yard or House Work.. 114

    Kegels 114

Join a Support Group... 115

Stop Smoking.. 116

Prioritize Sleep 117

To Summarize 118

CONCLUSION **119**

REFERENCES **123**

Introduction

Menopause is a word that can strike fear into the heart of many women, as it symbolizes a significant transition in their lives. It's often accompanied by uncomfortable symptoms such as hot flashes, mood swings, and feeling out of control. However, what if I told you menopause could also be a time of profound personal growth and new beginnings? It's a moment to embrace and adapt to your body's and life's transformations. As you navigate this chapter of your life, you can emerge stronger, more resilient, and self-assured. The central message of this book revolves around this empowering perspective on menopause.

In the pages that lie ahead, the various aspects of menopause will be explored, providing valuable advice to guide you through this significant phase of life. Menopause can be both challenging and exciting, and the aim is to support you every step of the way. The topics covered will range from the physical changes that occur during menopause to the emotional rollercoaster experienced by many women. In addition, comprehensive insights will be provided to help you understand and manage these transformations effectively.

However, menopause extends far beyond the physical realm. The emotional rollercoaster experienced during this time is equally important to address. Mood swings, anxiety, and depression will be explored, offering practical advice and strategies to navigate these emotional changes with grace and resilience. The goal is to empower you with the knowledge and tools to manage your emotional well-being during this transformative phase.

Self-care takes center stage as a critical component in navigating menopause with confidence and grace. Proper self-care encompasses tending to your physical, emotional, and spiritual needs. Prioritizing restful sleep, nourishing your body with a healthy and balanced diet, and engaging in regular exercise to promote overall well-being is essential. In addition, the significance of building a support network will be emphasized through connecting with support groups or seeking guidance from health-care providers.

While menopause encompasses a range of physical and emotional changes, this book goes beyond the surface to delve into the spiritual and psychological dimensions of this transformative phase. Menopause is an opportunity for self-discovery, growth, and embracing new possibilities. By exploring these dimensions, the aim is to inspire and motivate you to embark on a journey of self-exploration, unlocking your true potential and finding renewed meaning and purpose in this chapter of your life.

In essence, this book serves as a comprehensive roadmap, guiding you through the exciting and sometimes challenging terrain of menopause. Whether you're experiencing menopause symptoms for the first time or have been on this journey for quite a while, you will find valuable guidance, support, and motivation within these pages. So, sit back, grab a fan, pour yourself an ice-cold glass of water, and get ready to embark on an empowering journey of embracing and navigating menopause with confidence, optimism, and a renewed sense of purpose.

Chapter 1:

An Overview of

Menopause

This first chapter will delve into the fundamental aspects of this transformative phase in a woman's life. Menopause signifies the conclusion of the reproductive years and results in notable shifts in hormonal equilibrium, causing diverse physical and emotional symptoms.

In the following few pages, we will explore the definition of menopause, the three stages of menopause, and the common signs and symptoms accompanying this natural transition. By gaining a comprehensive understanding of menopause, you will be better equipped to navigate this chapter of your life with knowledge, confidence, and empowered decision-making.

Menopause Explained

Menopause is typically defined as the point in time when women have gone 12 consecutive months without experiencing a menstrual cycle. While some women may experience no significant symptoms during menopause, the transition can be accompanied by a range of discomforts for others. These may include hot flashes, insomnia, pain during intercourse, mood swings, irritability, and depression.

Women experiencing symptoms like hot flashes or irregular menstrual cycles may be entering the first stage of menopause, even if they don't realize it yet. Therefore, it's essential to recognize that menopause occurs in three stages, and consulting with a health-care provider can help clarify any uncertainty regarding the stage of menopause an individual is experiencing.

The Three Stages of Menopause

Perimenopause

The time before menopause is called perimenopause. During this period, women may observe changes in their menstrual cycles and encounter symptoms like hot flashes. It's important to note that perimenopause can last several years before menopause is reached, and seeking medical advice to manage any associated discomforts can be beneficial.

Perimenopause typically begins approximately 8–10 years before menopause, as the ovaries produce less estrogen. The phase known as perimenopause typically starts in a person's 40s and lasts until menopause, when the ovaries stop releasing eggs. During the final 1–2 years of perimenopause, the decline in estrogen production speeds up, resulting in several symptoms related to menopause. Despite this, it's important to note that menstruation still occurs during this stage, and individuals can still conceive and become pregnant.

Menopause

Menopause is when women permanently stop experiencing menstrual periods due to the ovaries ceasing to release eggs and produce estrogen. Menopause is usually diagnosed by health-care providers when a person has not had a menstrual period for 12 consecutive months.

Postmenopause

Postmenopause is the period that occurs after a person has gone through a whole year without experiencing a menstrual cycle or for the rest of their life after menopause. As menopause progresses, hot flashes and other symptoms may decrease, but some people may still experience them for over a decade after the transition. In addition, as estrogen levels decline after menopause, individuals may face higher risks for health issues such as osteoporosis and heart disease. During this time, eating a healthy diet, exercising regularly, and getting enough calcium to maintain optimal bone health is essential.

Other Possibilities

If you're experiencing symptoms commonly associated with menopause, your doctor may inquire about your symptoms, age, and family medical history to determine whether menopause is the root cause of your concerns. Sometimes, your doctor may suggest getting a blood test to check your follicle-stimulating hormone (FSH) and estradiol (E2) levels. This is done to eliminate any other possible reasons for your symptoms.

Menopause can also occur due to a hysterectomy or if you've had your ovaries, which are responsible for hormone production, surgically removed. If you've had your uterus or ovaries removed and don't take hormone replacement therapy (HRT), you'll experience menopausal symptoms right away.

Signs and Symptoms of Menopause

Throughout the transition to menopause, fluctuating hormone levels can impact your menstrual cycle, affecting your overall health. In addition, as you approach menopause, you may experience symptoms such as pain during sex, mood changes, and memory issues. It's essential to be aware of the signs and symptoms of menopause to prepare for and manage the changes that will happen.

Hot Flashes

The most prevalent symptom of menopause is hot flashes, which affect up to three out of four women. However, according to Shifren and Gass (2014), some women can experience hot flashes while still getting their period before menopause.

Hot flashes are sudden feelings of warmth that usually affect the upper body. During a hot flash, you may experience redness in your face and neck and red blotches on your chest, back, and arms. Heavy sweating is also common; some women may experience cold chills following a hot flash.

Research shows that hot flashes can continue for up to 14 years after menopause, although they are most frequent in the year before and after menopause (Avis et al., 2015; Tepperet al., 2016). However, despite the fact that the underlying reason for hot flashes during menopause is still not entirely understood, there are drugs that can help prevent some of them and management techniques for when they do occur.

Reduce Body Fat

It's common for women who are overweight or obese to experience more severe hot flashes. One study suggests that losing excess weight may be beneficial in alleviating hot flashes (Huang et al., 2010).

Keep Track of Your Hot Flashes

Consider noting the causes of your hot flashes and try to avoid them. For example, potential triggers could involve being in a warm environment, experiencing stress, or consuming caffeine, alcohol, or spicy foods. Keeping a record of what triggers your hot flashes will help you identify patterns and make lifestyle adjustments accordingly.

Practice Deep Breathing

When experiencing a hot flash, try to take slow and deep breaths. Doing so can signal your body to become calm and relaxed, potentially reducing the hot flash's duration.

Drink Cold Water

Drinking cold water can be a helpful way to lower your body temperature, relieving the discomfort of hot flashes. Keep a bottle of cold water nearby to take sips when you feel a hot flash coming on.

Use Fans

Using a fan can help you feel more comfortable during hot flashes. Consider keeping a small portable fan in your purse or bag to use whenever you feel a hot flash coming on. Placing a fan next to your bed at night and having one nearby at work is also a good idea.

Shed a Layer of Clothing

Dress in layers as much as possible. If you start feeling hot, you can remove a layer and put it back on when you feel cooler.

Use Hormones

Menopausal hormone therapy is a viable option for women who are experiencing menopause and are having hot flashes and night sweats. It can provide relief. However, if you're still menstruating, it's worth asking your doctor about low-dose hormonal birth control as a possible solution for your symptoms.

It's crucial to understand that this therapy carries certain risks. Before starting, discuss with your doctor whether it's right for you. If you decide to proceed with menopausal hormone therapy, aim to take the lowest effective dose for the shortest duration possible.

Use Other Medications

If you cannot have hormone treatments, discuss with your doctor the possibility of prescription medications usually prescribed for other medical conditions. For example, some antidepressants, blood-pressure medications, and epilepsy drugs may provide relief from hot flashes, even if you don't have these conditions.

Changes in Mood

Mood swings, including sudden crying spells or feelings of irritability, may occur during menopause. In addition, one study found that women who experienced mood changes during their monthly periods or postpartum depression may be more prone to mood changes during menopause as well (Roberts & Hickey, 2016).

Mood changes during menopause can happen to anyone, regardless of whether they had similar experiences during their menstrual cycle or after childbirth. Stress, fatigue, or family changes could trigger these mood changes. It's important to note that mood changes are different from depression.

To assist you in managing mood changes, here are some valuable tips:

- If you're experiencing mild mood changes due to menopause, it may be helpful to discuss menopausal hormone therapy with your doctor or nurse. All medicines have risks, including menopausal hormone therapy. It's important to note that the mood changes experienced during menopause are not the same as depression. Depression is a separate, serious illness that requires treatment.

- Join a support group in your local community or online, where you can connect with other women also going through menopause.

- Avoid taking on too many responsibilities and find ways to manage your stress positively.

- Find ways to get active to help you feel your best.

- Aim for 7–8 hours of sleep per night.

Memory Issues

It's common for women going through perimenopause to experience forgetfulness or difficulty concentrating. According to one study, up to two-thirds of women report experiencing these symptoms during this transitional phase (Weber et al., 2012). Furthermore, the study suggests that depression and lack of sleep are related to memory problems, but hormone estrogen levels are not.

If you want to enhance your memory, there are numerous tactics you can experiment with:

- Ensure to get enough sleep and physical activity, eat a healthy diet, and avoid smoking. These lifestyle factors help boost your memory.

- Stay socially active by joining a group or club that focuses on activities you enjoy, such as hiking or quilting. Social interaction has been linked to delayed memory loss and a lower risk of dementia and Alzheimer's disease.

- Keep your mind active by doing mental activities like crossword puzzles, taking classes, or learning a new language. These activities help improve your memory and concentration.

- If forgetfulness or other cognitive problems affect your daily life, ask your doctor for advice and guidance.

Anxiety and Depression

During menopause, you may be at higher risk for depression and anxiety due to menopausal symptoms, changing hormones, or both. In addition, the loss of fertility or changes in your body may cause feelings of sadness or depression. If you're experiencing symptoms of depression or anxiety, it's crucial to seek advice from your doctor. They may recommend therapy, medication, or a combination of both to help treat your symptoms. You can also try the following tactics:

- **Lessen stress:** Manage your stress by setting boundaries, practicing relaxation techniques, reading, spending time outdoors, or finding other healthy ways to unwind.

- **Lower alc0hol consumption:** Don't worry; there's no need to put the wine glasses away, but you'll have to track how much you're drinking. To maintain a healthy lifestyle, limit your alcohol consumption to one drink per day and no more than seven drinks per week. It's important to avoid binge drinking, which involves consuming more than four drinks in one sitting.

- **Exercise:** Including at least 30 minutes of physical activity in your daily routine for most days of the week is recommended. Research has demonstrated that engaging in physical activity can positively affect depression and anxiety symptoms (Singh et al., 2023).

- **Sleep:** Insufficient sleep is closely associated with depression. Therefore, it's crucial to ensure you obtain enough high-quality sleep. Strive for a duration of 7–8 hours of sleep per night.

Sleep Troubles

During menopause, some women may experience difficulty getting a good night's sleep due to hormonal changes. Specifically, low levels of progesterone can cause insomnia, while low estrogen levels can lead to hot flashes and night sweats that disrupt sleep.

Employ Good Sleep Habits

Create a restful sleep environment by keeping your bedroom cool, quiet, and dark. Reserve your bedroom for sleeping and sex, if possible. It's crucial to have a consistent sleep schedule by going to bed and waking up at the same time every day. If you experience difficulty sleeping at night, try doing some calming activities until you feel tired again.

Consult Your Doctor

If you're experiencing difficulty sleeping, discussing your sleep problems with your doctor is crucial, as it could indicate a severe issue. In addition, sleep apnea or insomnia are common conditions for women going through menopause, and treating sleep problems can also aid in improving chronic pain.

Exercise

Incorporating exercise into your daily routine can significantly enhance the quality of your sleep. Starting to exercise during menopause, even if you haven't done it before, can help you feel better. In addition, you may want to consider specific exercises like stretching and yoga, which have been found to improve hot flashes (Innes et al., 2010). However, avoid exercising too close to bedtime as it may make you more alert instead of sleepy.

Explore Options for Managing Hot Flashes

If hot flashes keep you awake at night, discussing treatment options with your doctor or nurse is advisable. Treating hot flashes will usually improve your sleep.

Address Bladder Problems

Urinary or bladder incontinence is not a normal part of the aging process. Therefore, you should talk to your doctor if you experience it. There are many treatment options for any urinary issues.

Don't Smoke, Drink Alcohol, or Eat Before Bed

Avoid large meals, smoking, and drinking alcohol right before bedtime. Also, avoid caffeine after noon.

Consume Warm Drinks

Try drinking something warm before bedtime, such as caffeine-free tea or warm milk.

Limit Screen-Time

Limit TV, phone, or computer use near bedtime, especially in your bedroom. The bright light of the screens tells your brain to wake up instead of sleep.

Changed Attitude Toward Sex

Following menopause, some women may feel more at ease with their sexuality, while others may experience decreased sexual arousal. Discomfort or pain during sexual activity may reduce interest in sex. Vaginal tissue may become thinner and drier, leading to discomfort or pain during sexual intercourse.

Some women may experience a decreased interest in sex during menopause due to symptoms like depression, anxiety, or lack of sleep. If you're experiencing adverse effects from menopause symptoms, discussing potential treatments with your doctor is essential.

If vaginal dryness is causing discomfort, safe over-the-counter and prescription treatments are available to improve vaginal lubrication. In addition, it's essential to be informed about menopause and how it can affect your sexuality.

Irregular Bleeding and Periods

Your periods' frequency, duration, and flow may change during perimenopause. However, missing a few periods does not necessarily indicate that you're in the transition to menopause.

It's essential to consult your doctor to rule out other reasons for missed periods, such as pregnancy or underlying health issues. For example, if you experience vaginal spotting or bleeding after not having a period for a year, you may have a severe health condition like cancer, and you should seek medical attention immediately.

Vaginal Complications

During menopause, you may experience vaginal problems such as dryness that can lead to itching, burning, pain, and discomfort due to the low estrogen levels in your body. This can also make sexual intercourse painful and cause minor cuts and tears in your vaginal tissue, which increases your risk of getting sexually transmitted infections (STIs) (Muhleisen & Herbst-Kralovetz, 2016). Thankfully, you can take steps to avoid vaginal infections and related issues.

Prescription Medicine

Consult with your health-care provider to explore alternative methods of treating vaginal dryness, such as prescription estrogen creams, gels, low-dose hormonal birth control, or vaginal rings. Learning more about these treatments and understanding the risks involved is essential, so be sure to have a conversation with your doctor first.

Vaginal Lubricant

To make sex more comfortable, you can use a water-based vaginal lubricant that can be purchased over the counter. This should be applied before or during sex.

Vaginal Moisturizer

Using an over-the-counter vaginal moisturizer every few days can help maintain lubrication and increase comfort during sexual activity. However, it's vital to select a vaginal moisturizer that's free from perfumes and dyes to avoid irritation and worsening of symptoms.

Urinary Issues

Urinary issues, such as bladder weakness or incontinence, are common among women in menopause. The decrease in estrogen levels can result in weakened urethra muscles, leading to urinary urge or stress incontinence. For instance, some women may experience urine leakage when laughing, sneezing, or coughing. Moreover, the need to urinate during sleep can disrupt your sleep quality. However, it's important to remember that urinary problems are not a regular aspect of getting older and can be remedied.

Various treatment options are available for urinary incontinence, depending on the underlying cause. These may include surgery, physical therapy, using specialized medical devices, taking medication, and avoiding or limiting caffeine.

If you experience urine leakage, there are products available such as a pessary, a urethra cap, or pads. A pessary is a circular disk inserted into your vagina to support your bladder, while a urethra cap fits over your urinary opening and can be reused. Your doctor will assist you in finding the right fit for your pessary.

Afterward, you can clean and reinsert it yourself. Your doctor can also suggest various methods you can try at home to help manage urinary incontinence. These may include losing weight to alleviate pressure on your bladder or Kegels, which are pelvic floor muscle exercises.

To Summarize

Throughout this chapter, we've covered what menopause is and the three stages of menopause: perimenopause, menopause, and postmenopause. We've also explored the various symptoms that women may experience during menopause and some possible solutions for those symptoms.

The next chapter will dive more deeply into menopause treatments, including hormonal and non-hormonal options. Additionally, we will discuss the hormonal changes that occur during menopause and why menopause happens. This information will help you make informed decisions about your health and well-being throughout this critical life transition.

Chapter 2:

Hormonal Changes During

Menopause

Now that you understand menopause's signs and symptoms, let's explore its causes and treatment options. First, we'll delve into the biological processes behind menopause, such as the decline in reproductive hormones and ovulation cessation. Additionally, we'll discuss a range of treatment approaches. This chapter will provide you with valuable insights and practical strategies to confidently navigate this transformative phase.

The Cause of Menopause

Natural menopause is a part of the aging process where your reproductive cycle begins to slow down and ultimately ceases. This cycle has been functioning continuously since puberty. The leading cause of menopause is reduced hormone levels produced by the ovaries, specifically estrogen and progesterone.

Estrogen

The hormone estrogen is essential for the proper functioning of a woman's reproductive system. The ovaries primarily produce it, but the adrenal glands and fat cells can also make it.

During menopause, levels of estrogen decrease as the ovaries stop producing it. This hormonal change can cause various symptoms, such as hot flashes, night sweats, vaginal dryness, mood changes, and decreased bone density. However, estrogen also helps to maintain healthy skin, hair, and vaginal tissue, promotes bone growth and strength, and helps maintain healthy cholesterol levels. Estrogen has also been shown to have neuroprotective effects, which may help protect against cognitive decline and Alzheimer's disease.

Hormone therapy involving estrogen has been controversial due to its potential risks, which include an increased risk of blood clots, stroke, and breast cancer. Therefore, discussing hormone therapy's potential benefits and risks with a health-care provider is essential.

Progesterone

In the female reproductive system, progesterone is a vital hormone produced by the ovaries. Its primary role is to prepare the uterus for pregnancy. During a typical menstrual cycle, levels of progesterone increase after ovulation and stay elevated for approximately 2 weeks. However, progesterone levels drop if pregnancy doesn't occur, and the menstrual cycle starts again.

During menopause, the ovaries produce less progesterone. Changes in the menstrual cycle, like missed or irregular periods, can result from this. Progesterone is also involved in many physical and emotional symptoms women experience during menopause, including hot flashes, mood swings, and sleep disturbances.

Progesterone therapy, either alone or in combination with estrogen, may be used to treat menopausal symptoms. Progesterone therapy is usually recommended only for women who have undergone a hysterectomy and therefore do not require protection against the risk of uterine cancer associated with estrogen therapy. Before beginning hormone therapy, weighing the potential advantages and disadvantages is essential.

Treating Menopause

If you're experiencing menopause symptoms, it's essential to know that not all women require treatment. Sometimes, symptoms can disappear independently or may not bother you enough to seek treatment. However, if you're uncomfortable or struggling to cope with your symptoms, don't hesitate to talk to your doctor. You can explore ways to relieve your symptoms and improve your quality of life. For some women, making lifestyle changes like increasing physical activity and adjusting their diet can be helpful, while others may benefit from medication or other treatments. Discovering a solution that suits you and promotes your overall health and well-being is crucial.

Medicines for Menopause

Hormone Therapy

Menopausal hormone therapy is a prescription medication used to alleviate severe menopause symptoms, such as vaginal dryness and hot flashes that interfere with your daily routine. This therapy can be referred to as HRT or hormone therapy.

In menopause, the ovaries produce significantly lower levels of estrogen and progesterone hormones. Menopausal hormone therapy substitutes the lost hormones with synthetic estrogen and progesterone. Menopausal hormone therapy is available in various forms, including oral pills taken once a day or a skin patch containing estrogen, progesterone, or both. Unfortunately, menopausal hormone therapy isn't safe for all women, so discussing any risks with your doctor is crucial.

When considering your health, it's crucial to consider particular factors such as a history of heart disease or risk factors like high cholesterol and any personal or family history of breast cancer. Other factors to consider include high levels of triglycerides in your blood, a family history of gallbladder disease, liver disease, and a history of stroke or blood clots. It's crucial to understand that menopausal hormone therapy might not be the most suitable choice for women with these risk factors.

It's essential to mention that taking estrogen alone or with progesterone increases the chances of developing blood clots in the lungs and legs, as well as the risk of stroke. These risks are rare in women between 50 and 59. Menopausal hormone therapy may be a safe option for women up to age 59, but usually only within 10 years of menopause. Women who are younger or closer to their final menstrual period may experience fewer adverse effects.

With all these risks in mind, it's understandable that the U.S. Food and Drug Administration (FDA) advises women who want to try menopausal hormone therapy to use the lowest effective dose for the shortest duration possible.

Risks aside, there is also an abundance of benefits. The North American Menopause Society (2014) states menopausal hormone therapy can help reduce menopause symptoms, such as vaginal dryness, mood changes, sleep problems, and hot flashes. It's worth noting that hot flashes typically require higher doses of estrogen therapy, which affects your entire body.

Topical vaginal estrogen can also be used if you experience vaginal discomfort or dryness during sex. Another FDA-approved medication to alleviate painful sex due to vaginal dryness after menopause is a hormonal medicine called prasterone. This medication is applied once a day inside the vagina.

Selective Estrogen Receptor Modulators

Selective estrogen receptor modulators (SERMs) are hormone therapies that regulate estrogen in the body. Medications like raloxifene and tamoxifen belong to this category and have proven efficacy in treating specific breast cancer types and osteoporosis.

Health-care providers commonly prescribe tamoxifen for women who have not yet experienced menopause. However, for women who have already experienced menopause and are at an increased risk of developing breast cancer, raloxifene may be recommended as a treatment.

SERMs have diverse medical roles. They function by inhibiting estrogen from binding to breast cancer cells, effectively preventing their proliferation. Concurrently, SERMs mimic the effects of estrogen by increasing estrogen levels in the bones, thus aiding in the prevention of osteoporosis.

Strontium Ranelate

Strontium ranelate is a medication that has been used in the treatment of osteoporosis. It's a synthetic compound that combines the element strontium with ranelic acid. Strontium is thought to have bone-strengthening properties and is believed to promote new bone formation while inhibiting bone resorption.

The drug has been used to decrease the likelihood of fractures in women who have gone through menopause and are experiencing osteoporosis. Research has shown that using 2 g of strontium ranelate daily over a period of 3 years can effectively reduce fractures in the spine and slightly decrease fractures in other areas in postmenopausal women with osteoporosis (Adachi et al., 2006).

Most women who use strontium ranelate do not experience significant side effects that would lead them to discontinue its use. However, further research has revealed possible dangers, including an elevated risk of blood clots and seizures and potential impacts on memory and consciousness (O'Donnell et al., 2006).

It's important to note that strontium ranelate is unavailable in some countries and may have certain restrictions or warnings associated with its use. Therefore, if you're considering using strontium ranelate, seeking advice from your health-care provider is crucial. They can offer guidance and help clarify the potential benefits and risks involved.

Bisphosphonates

Bisphosphonates are medications used to treat osteoporosis by blocking bone resorption. Doing so helps preserve or even enhance bone mineral density and contributes to maintaining bone architecture. Unfortunately, women who have reached menopause and have osteoporosis, particularly those who have experienced a fracture, face a higher risk of future fractures. This is attributed to the decline in bone mineral density and the deterioration of bone structure.

An analysis of multiple studies revealed that women undergoing bisphosphonate therapy experienced a notable reduction in the risk of future fractures (Imam et al., 2019). Furthermore, the review indicated a significant increase in bone mineral density among those receiving bisphosphonate treatment. These findings suggest that bisphosphonate therapy can effectively enhance bone mineral density and reduce the likelihood of future fractures. However, more research is needed to determine the specific increase in bone mineral density that would effectively lower the chances of experiencing future fractures.

Low-Dose Hormonal Birth Control

As you approach menopause, taking low-dose hormonal birth control can help relieve symptoms like mood swings, vaginal dryness, hot flashes, and irregular or heavy periods. If you smoke, it's better to steer clear of hormonal birth control as it can raise the chances of blood clots and high blood pressure. This is particularly true for combination skin patches, vaginal rings, and birth control pills.

Bioidentical Hormone Therapy

"Bioidentical" is a term used by manufacturers of bioidentical hormone therapy to imply that their products are similar to natural hormones. In addition, several of these companies assert that their products pose fewer risks than menopausal hormone therapy.

Nonetheless, the FDA neither regulates these products nor recognizes this term, and no studies have been done to evaluate their effectiveness or safety. Therefore, before trying any bioidentical hormone therapy, it's advisable to consult your doctor.

Antidepressants

Antidepressants are medications designed to alleviate symptoms associated with depression by targeting neurotransmitters, which facilitate communication between brain cells. Contrary to their name, antidepressants are not limited to treating depression alone. They can effectively address various conditions, including anxiety and panic disorders, insomnia, chronic pain, eating disorders, and migraines. Moreover, antidepressants have been explored as a potential treatment for menopause symptoms. Antidepressants can alleviate vasomotor symptoms associated with menopause, which primarily involve the blood vessels and include hot flashes, skin flushing, and night sweats.

Research indicates that using low doses of selective serotonin reuptake inhibitors (SSRIs) or serotonin–norepinephrine reuptake inhibitors (SNRIs) can be beneficial in diminishing vasomotor symptoms, particularly hot flashes and night sweats. For instance, a clinical trial demonstrated that a low dose of the SNRI venlafaxine (Effexor) yielded comparable results to conventional hormone therapy in reducing the frequency and intensity of hot flashes (Joffe et al., 2014).

In a separate clinical trial, it was observed that a low dose of the SSRI paroxetine (Paxil) enhanced the quality of sleep among menopausal women. The improvement was due to the participants experiencing fewer nighttime vasomotor symptoms while taking paroxetine (Pinkerton et al., 2015).

While the outcomes of these tests are promising, it's still unclear how SSRIs and SNRIs relieve vasomotor symptoms. It's hypothesized that their ability to regulate norepinephrine and serotonin levels may play a role. These neurotransmitters are involved in temperature regulation in the body.

It's noteworthy that antidepressants can effectively alleviate hot flashes and night sweats. However, if you're seeking treatment for other menopause symptoms, hormone therapy may be a more suitable and effective option.

While antidepressants are generally considered safe, it's important to note that the use of most antidepressants for managing menopause symptoms is considered "off label." This means that the manufacturers of these antidepressants have not conducted extensive trials to establish their safety and effectiveness specifically for treating hot flashes and night sweats.

Additionally, antidepressants may interact with other medications. Therefore, when considering antidepressants, you must inform your doctor about all of the over-the-counter and prescription drugs, vitamins, and supplements you're taking. In addition, it's essential to tell your doctor of any medical conditions or risk factors you may have, such as glaucoma, a history of heart disease, high cholesterol, or an increased risk of heart attack or stroke. Sharing this information with your doctor will help them evaluate the benefits and risks of using antidepressants for managing menopause symptoms. Your doctor can then provide you with appropriate guidance.

Pregabalin and Gabapentin

Pregabalin and gabapentin are medications that exert their effects on the brain. Gabapentin is primarily prescribed for seizures and nerve pain associated with conditions like herpes. It's also used to manage anxiety, insomnia, and mood disorders. Pregabalin is commonly used to alleviate fibromyalgia pain, seizures, nerve pain, and anxiety. Due to their impact on the brain, these medications have been the subject of research regarding their potential effects on menopause symptoms.

Pregabalin is primarily used for women with both fibromyalgia and bothersome menopausal symptoms. However, it's essential to note that pregabalin is relatively more expensive than gabapentin and may adversely affect platelets and muscle function.

On the other hand, for women experiencing night sweats, hot flashes, physical discomfort, and sleep disturbances, gabapentin may be a viable option to consider. The risks associated with gabapentin are generally low, and the side effects are minimal when using the low doses typically prescribed for these symptoms. Treatment typically begins with a low amount that is gradually increased. It's advisable to take gabapentin at bedtime to benefit from its drowsiness side effect, which can aid sleep.

Approximately 10% of individuals who take gabapentin or pregabalin report experiencing dizziness and drowsiness as side effects. Additionally, a few women may experience sexual dysfunction, including a loss of libido and difficulty achieving orgasm, when using these medications. Other possible side effects associated with gabapentin and pregabalin include confusion, blurred or double vision, euphoria, headaches, slurred speech, tingling sensations, vertigo, vivid dreams, tremors, unsteady gait, gastrointestinal discomfort, weight gain, memory impairment, dry mouth, irritability, and peripheral edema.

Topical Vaginal Estrogen

Vaginal estrogen belongs to a group of medications known as hormones. Its mechanism of action involves replacing the natural estrogen typically produced by the body. This treatment is available for women who have gone through or are currently experiencing menopause and are dealing with symptoms like vaginal dryness, itching, and burning. It can also help alleviate issues like painful or difficult urination and a sudden urgent need to urinate.

Vaginal estrogen is available in different forms for administration. In addition, various options for birth control can be used inside the vagina, such as a flexible ring, vaginal insert, tablet, or cream. Estrogen vaginal rings are typically inserted into the vagina and can remain in place for up to3 months. After 3 months, the ring is removed, and a new one can be inserted if continued treatment is required.

Vaginal estrogen inserts are typically used once daily at the same time for 2 weeks, followed by a maintenance dose of once every 3–4 days (twice weekly) as needed. Estrogen vaginal tablets are usually inserted once a day for the initial 2 weeks of treatment and then twice a week for as long as treatment is necessary.

It's essential to use vaginal estrogen at approximately the same time each day as instructed. In addition, it's vital to follow the directions on your prescription label. If you have difficulty comprehending anything, don't hesitate to seek assistance from your doctor or pharmacist. Finally, use vaginal estrogen precisely as prescribed, avoiding excess or insufficient amounts, and refrain from using it more frequently than your doctor directs.

If you're experiencing persistent or severe side effects from vaginal estrogen, it's essential to inform your doctor as soon as possible. These side effects include:

- swelling, redness, burning, itching, or irritation of the vagina

- back or joint pain

- nausea

- headache

- stomach pain or bloating

- changes in sexual desire

- diarrhea

- vomiting

- hair loss

- painful or difficult urination

- breast pain or tenderness

- sudden feelings of heat or sweating

- difficulty falling asleep or staying asleep

- runny nose or congestion

- spotty darkening of the skin on the face

- vaginal discharge

It's crucial to promptly contact your doctor if you encounter any of the following symptoms as they may indicate a severe condition:

- persistent pain originating in the abdominal area and spreading to the back

- episodes of nausea

- vomiting, or a noticeable decrease in appetite

- bulging eyes

- the development of a rash, hives, or itching

- experiencing hoarseness, difficulty breathing, or swallowing difficulties

- swelling in the lower legs, ankles, feet, arms, hands, throat, tongue, eyes, or face

- the presence of fever, nausea or vomiting, diarrhea, muscle pain, dizziness, or fainting

- a rash on the face or body

Over-the-Counter Products

There are products available without a prescription, commonly known as over-the-counter (OTC) products, that can help alleviate symptoms of vaginal discomfort, dryness, or pain. For example, a water-based vaginal lubricant can help make sex more comfortable. In addition, a vaginal moisturizer can help keep needed moisture in vaginal tissues and make sex more comfortable.

To Summarize

Understanding the hormonal changes during menopause, exploring various treatment options, and incorporating exercise into your daily routine can empower you to manage menopause more confidently. In addition, by staying informed about the changes happening in your body and seeking professional guidance, you can make informed decisions regarding hormone therapy, medications, and alternative treatments to alleviate troublesome symptoms.

In the next chapter, we'll discuss HRT. In the upcoming pages, we'll delve into the intricacies of HRT, exploring its benefits, potential risks, and important considerations.

Chapter 3:

Hormone Replacement

Therapy

In this chapter, we dive into the intriguing world of HRT. HRT is a popular topic of discussion and debate when treating menopause symptoms, and it's essential to weigh its risks and benefits carefully. As such, we will explore HRT's potential advantages and drawbacks, shedding light on its effectiveness in managing menopausal symptoms. Additionally, we will delve into the controversies surrounding HRT and provide guidelines to help you make informed decisions about its use. So, get ready to explore the complexities of HRT as you're guided through its intricacies, giving you the knowledge needed to make informed decisions for your well-being.

An Overview of Hormone

Replacement Therapy

HRT involves using medication that contains female hormones to supplement the declining estrogen levels during menopause. Its primary purpose is alleviating common menopausal symptoms such as vaginal discomfort and hot flashes. Furthermore, HRT has been proven to reduce fracture risk and prevent bone loss among postmenopausal women.

Nevertheless, it's essential to know the risks associated with HRT. These risks depend on factors such as the specific type of hormone therapy, dosage, duration of medication use, and individual health considerations. For the best results, HRT should be tailored to each person and monitored regularly to ensure the advantages outweigh possible drawbacks.

Risks and Benefits of Hormone Replacement Therapy

Several factors can affect the risks and benefits of HRT, including the type of hormones used, dosage, duration of use, and individual health characteristics. Therefore, it's essential to consider all of these factors when weighing the pros and cons of HRT.

Risks and Considerations of Hormone Replacement Therapy

Increased Risk of Blood Clots

HRT, particularly when taken orally, can raise the risk of blood clot formation, including deep-vein thrombosis and pulmonary embolism. Older women, individuals with a history of blood clots, and smokers are at a higher risk. Transdermal (patch or gel) administration may be less risky than oral administration.

Endometrial Cancer Risk

It's important to note that women with uteruses who take estrogen-only therapy have a higher risk of developing endometrial cancer. However, adding progestin to estrogen therapy significantly reduces this risk by protecting the lining of the uterus (endometrium).

Potential Increase in Breast Cancer Risk

Long-term use of combined estrogen and progestin therapy (for women with a uterus) may slightly increase the risk of developing breast cancer. Estrogen-only therapy (for women who have had a hysterectomy) may lower the risk of breast cancer. The increased risk, if present, tends to be minor and dependent on the duration and specific type of HRT used.

Stroke Risk

According to some studies, older women who undergo oral estrogen therapy may have a slightly higher risk of stroke (Lisabeth & Bushnell, 2012; Henderson & Lobo, 2012). In addition, the risk may be higher for women with other risk factors, such as a history of cardiovascular disease, high blood pressure, or if they smoke. On the other hand, transdermal administration of estrogen may carry a lower stroke risk than oral administration.

Individual Health Factors

The risks and benefits of HRT can vary depending on individual health factors. For example, women with a history of ovarian or breast cancer, liver disease, blood clotting disorders, or certain cardiovascular conditions may have higher risks associated with HRT. Therefore, discussing personal medical history and evaluating individual risks with a health-care professional is crucial.

Benefits of Hormone Replacement Therapy

Relief for Menopausal Symptoms

HRT effectively reduces common menopausal symptoms like hot flashes, night sweats, and vaginal dryness. By providing the body with hormones it no longer produces in sufficient amounts, HRT can alleviate these discomforts and improve overall quality of life during menopause.

Improved Quality of Life

Menopausal symptoms can significantly impact daily life, causing sleep disturbances, mood changes, and decreased well-being. HRT can help manage these symptoms, promoting better sleep, stabilizing mood, and enhancing overall quality of life.

Prevention of Bone Loss

Maintaining bone density is crucial, and estrogen is responsible for this. However, during menopause, the decline in estrogen increases the risk of osteoporosis and fractures. HRT with estrogen can slow down bone loss, reduce the risk of fractures, and help maintain bone health in postmenopausal women.

Potential Cardiovascular Benefits

Initiating hormone therapy within a specific time frame after menopause may have cardiovascular benefits. Estrogen can positively affect cholesterol levels, arterial health, and blood vessel function, reducing the risk of heart disease. However, the cardiovascular effects of HRT can vary based on individual factors and should be carefully evaluated and discussed with a health-care provider.

When considering HRT, it's crucial to make your decision based on a thorough evaluation of your personal risks and preferences. Therefore, before deciding to take HRT, it's advisable to consult a healthcare provider with expertise in this field. In addition, regular reevaluation of the benefits and risks is recommended to ensure that the chosen approach is most appropriate for each person's circumstances.

Controversy Surrounding Hormone Replacement Therapy

There are several controversies surrounding menopause that have sparked ongoing discussions and debates among health-care professionals and researchers.

Hormone Replacement Therapy and Breast Cancer Risk

The association between HRT and breast cancer risk has been controversial. While some studies have suggested a slight increase in the risk of breast cancer with long-term use of combined estrogen and progestin therapy, other studies have reported conflicting results (Chlebowski et al., 2015; Vinogradova et al., 2020). The interpretation of these findings and the overall risk–benefit assessment of HRT concerning breast cancer remains a subject of debate.

Cardiovascular Effects of Hormone Therapy

The impact of hormone therapy on cardiovascular health has also been controversial. Earlier observational studies suggested potential cardiovascular benefits of HRT, while subsequent randomized controlled trials yielded different results (Warren & Halpert, 2004; Cagnacci & Venier, 2019). The inconsistent findings have led to ongoing discussions regarding the optimal timing, duration, and individualized approach to hormone therapy for cardiovascular health.

Alternatives to Hormone Therapy

The effectiveness and safety of alternative approaches to managing menopausal symptoms have been debated. As a result, some women turn to complementary and alternative therapies, such as herbal supplements, acupuncture, or mind–body practices, as alternatives to hormone therapy. Unfortunately, the proof of the effectiveness and safety of these alternatives is limited and often inconsistent.

Long-Term Effects of Early Menopause

Early menopause, either natural or surgical, raises concerns about potential long-term health consequences, including increased risks of cardiovascular disease, osteoporosis, cognitive decline, and overall mortality. The optimal management strategies for women who experience early menopause and the potential benefits of hormone therapy in this population are topics of ongoing research and discussion.

Individualized Approaches and Shared Decision-Making

Every woman's experience with menopause is unique, and management of its symptoms should be tailored to your specific needs. However, there is ongoing debate regarding the best methods for shared decision-making between health-care providers and women, considering their preferences, health history, and risk factors. Finding the proper balance between easing symptoms, assessing risks, and prioritizing the overall health of each woman can be challenging.

These controversies highlight the complexities and nuances involved in understanding and managing menopause. Ongoing research, advances in personalized medicine, and an improved understanding of individual risk factors will continue to shape the discussions and controversies surrounding menopause and its management.

Guidelines for Using Hormone Replacement Therapy

Use of HRT can vary based on individual factors, medical history, and specific symptoms. However, health-care professionals follow general recommendations and guidelines when prescribing HRT.

Individualized Approach

HRT should be individualized based on your unique circumstances, including age, menopausal stage, overall health, and specific symptoms. Treatment decisions should be made through shared decision-making between you and your health-care provider.

Symptom Severity and Impact

HRT primarily alleviates moderate to severe menopausal symptoms that significantly affect your quality of life. When considering HRT, common symptoms that are taken into account include hot flashes, night sweats, vaginal dryness, and mood changes.

Timing of Initiation

HRT is most effective when initiated closer to the onset of menopause or within the first 10 years after menopause. Early HRT initiation may result in greater symptom alleviation and perhaps bone and cardiovascular advantages.

Shortest Duration and Lowest Effective Dose

The general principle is to use the lowest effective dose of HRT for the shortest duration needed to alleviate symptoms. This approach helps minimize potential risks associated with long-term use of HRT.

Combination or Estrogen-Only Therapy

The decision to use combined estrogen–progestin or estrogen-only therapy depends on factors such as whether you still have your uterus. If so, you may require progestin and estrogen to protect against the increased risk of endometrial cancer.

Regular Reassessment

To assess the continued need for HRT, attending regular follow-up appointments with a health-care provider is crucial. In addition, periodic reassessment of symptoms, potential risks, and overall health status allows for adjustments in the treatment plan as necessary.

Individual Health Risks and Considerations

The decision to use HRT also involves considering individual health risks and factors. This includes evaluating your medical and family history and assessing HRT's potential benefits versus risks concerning conditions such as cardiovascular disease, breast cancer, stroke, blood clots, and osteoporosis.

It's important to note that these guidelines provide a general framework, and the specific recommendations for HRT can vary depending on the individual. For this reason, seeking guidance from a health-care expert who can evaluate your circumstances, suggest personalized strategies, and keep a close eye on your response to HRT is advised.

To Summarize

This chapter delved into the topic of HRT, providing an overview of its purpose and usage. We explored the potential risks and benefits associated with HRT, highlighting the importance of personalized evaluation and ongoing monitoring to ensure that the benefits outweigh the risks for each individual. Additionally, we discussed the controversies surrounding HRT, acknowledging the ongoing debates and evolving perspectives within the medical community.

In the upcoming chapter, we will provide helpful information about how supplements can effectively manage the challenges of this transitional phase of life and their potential benefits. Additionally, we will explore a range of supplements you may consider to alleviate your symptoms, examining the existing research to understand their efficacy and safety considerations.

Chapter 4:

Supplements for

Menopause

In this section, you will discover valuable information about the effectiveness of supplements in managing menopause symptoms. We will explore a range of supplements you may wish to consider to alleviate your symptoms.

Throughout the chapter, we will examine the existing research to help you understand the potential benefits, efficacy, and safety considerations associated with these supplements. The goal is to give you valuable information about how supplements can support you during this transitional phase of life. So, let's dive in!

Do Supplements Work?

The National Center for Complementary and Integrative Health (NCCIH) states that the effectiveness of dietary supplements in alleviating menopause symptoms is still uncertain (Dresden, 2021). While some women may find relief from specific symptoms by taking supplements, the overall impact and effectiveness are not yet fully understood or supported by strong scientific evidence.

It's important to note that the NCCIH emphasizes the limited research available on the long-term safety of these supplements. Therefore, further scientific investigation is necessary to better understand the potential benefits and risks of using dietary supplements for menopause symptoms.

Supplements for Managing Menopause Symptoms

Determining which supplements are the best for menopause symptoms is not as straightforward as you may think. Therefore, before initiating any vitamin or supplement regimens, it's crucial to consult your doctor. In addition, supplements are unregulated and can, thus, potentially lead to severe health issues such as liver toxicity. Just because a product is purchased from a health-food store does not guarantee safety.

Additionally, it's widely agreed that a nutritious and well-balanced diet is the most effective approach to ensure sufficient vitamin and mineral intake. However, in some instances, supplements may be recommended by a medical professional. For example, your doctor may advise you to take supplements during the menopausal period. Therefore, remember to carefully review warnings, labels, and dosage instructions, and, most importantly, seek your doctor's professional guidance.

Calcium

During menopause, bone loss becomes a concern, and maintaining adequate calcium levels is crucial for maintaining bone health. However, if you already consume a substantial amount of calcium-rich foods, such as dairy products and leafy greens, you may obtain sufficient calcium through your diet.

Obtaining calcium through your diet is preferable to relying on supplements. However, individuals who experience gastrointestinal problems or have lactose intolerance may find it challenging to get sufficient dietary calcium. The human body naturally contains calcium, with adult females typically having around 1,200 g of calcium until menopause, when estrogen levels decline. If you need more calcium from your diet and are of a certain age, your doctor may suggest taking a calcium supplement to ensure you reach the recommended daily intake of 1,000–1,200 mg.

A study conducted by LeBlanc et al. (2015) examined the impact of calcium and vitamin D supplements on menopausal symptoms. The participants were administered 1,000 mg of calcium and 400 international units (IU) of vitamin D throughout the study, and the researchers conducted follow-ups with the participants over an average period of 5.7 years.

The findings revealed no notable difference in symptoms between the group that did not receive supplements and the group that did. In addition, both groups' emotional well-being, energy levels, and sleep disturbances exhibited similar patterns, leading the researchers to conclude that calcium and vitamin D supplements are unlikely to influence menopausal symptoms.

Vitamin D

Vitamin D, called the "sunshine vitamin," is crucial for calcium absorption and overall health. While some individuals can obtain sufficient amounts through sun exposure and vitamin-D-rich foods, such as orange juice, dairy, fortified products, oily fish, and egg yolks, those approaching menopause may be at risk of deficiency.

Maintaining bone health is crucial, and vitamin D plays a critical role. It helps prevent osteoporosis, a condition where bone density decreases and bones become more fragile. Menopause-related hormonal changes can contribute to osteoporosis, particularly in susceptible individuals. For example, in the 5–7 years following menopause, some women may experience a significant reduction of up to one-fifth of their bone density. Therefore, ensuring adequate vitamin D and calcium intake during the menopausal period can help prevent the onset of osteoporosis.

The Office on Women's Health in the United States recommends a daily intake of 600 IU of vitamin D up to the age of 70 and an increased intake of 800 IU per day for individuals aged 71 and older ("Osteoporosis," 2021).

While the body creates a significant amount of vitamin D through sunlight exposure, some individuals use sunscreen or limit sun exposure to protect their skin. To assess whether supplementation is necessary, a doctor can perform a blood test to measure vitamin D levels.

Consult a doctor for guidance on the appropriate dosage and sources of vitamin D. It's worth noting that excessive vitamin D intake can potentially raise the risk of heart and kidney issues ("Vitamin D," 2022). Additionally, excessive vitamin D intake can lead to elevated calcium levels, which may be undesirable. Therefore, moderation is key.

Vitamin E

You can obtain vitamin E through various food sources, such as tomatoes, mangoes, kiwifruit, broccoli, spinach, sunflower seeds, and nuts. Vitamin E is an antioxidant that helps reduce oxidative stress in the body caused by an overabundance of free radicals. Free radicals can be generated due to various biological processes and environmental factors.

A research study showed that antioxidants could help protect the body from age-related illnesses like heart disease and cancer by preventing changes in the body that occur as we age (Phaniendra et al., 2014). However, another study indicated a potential association between diminished levels of antioxidants and depression and anxiety, which are everyday experiences during the menopausal transition (Xu et al., 2014).

Vitamin C

As an antioxidant, vitamin C has the potential to aid in the prevention of certain diseases that can arise due to oxidative stress, including specific forms of cardiovascular disease. Additionally, women who have a higher intake of vitamin C during menopause may potentially experience benefits such as higher bone density and better performance on cognitive tests compared with those with a lower intake, according to some studies (Milart et al., 2018). Vitamin C is vital in supporting the immune system and promoting collagen production, a fundamental component of skin and cellular structure.

Foods high in vitamin C include peppers, oranges, grapefruit, kiwifruit, broccoli, strawberries, Brussel sprouts, tomatoes, cantaloupe, cabbage, cauliflower, potatoes, spinach, and green peas.

B Vitamins

Specific individuals may find B vitamins beneficial during the menopausal period. One study emphasized the significant role of B vitamins, stating that their importance in menopause cannot be overstated (Milart et al., 2018). The study further highlighted that vitamin deficiency during this transitional phase could negatively affect health outcomes.

Adequate intake of B vitamins may play a role in reducing the risk of dementia, cardiovascular disease, stroke, and conditions that commonly affect older individuals and may manifest during menopause. Specifically, vitamins B_6 and B_{12} are believed to support cognitive function, including memory, reasoning, and thinking. Menopausal women often report experiencing a lack of focus, memory issues, and "brain fog." Therefore, ensuring sufficient levels of these vitamins may help lower the risk of developing dementia over time, regardless of menopausal status.

Additionally, evidence suggests that depression tends to be elevated during the menopausal transition (Clayton & Ninan, 2010). One study has indicated that consuming sufficient vitamin B_6 may reduce the risk of depression among older individuals, including those going through menopause (Gougeon et al., 2015).

Research has also indicated that individuals with low levels of vitamin B_2, B_6, and B_{12} may have decreased bone mineral density, a risk factor for osteoporosis. Additionally, research has shown that vitamin B_9, also known as folate, can effectively reduce the frequency and intensity of hot flashes experienced by individuals (Bani et al., 2013).

Here are some dietary sources of B vitamins:

- **B_{12}:** eggs, fish, chicken, dairy products, fortified nutritional yeasts, beef liver, and clams
- **B_9 (folate):** lettuce, asparagus, cereals, fortified breakfast cereals, black-eyed peas, spinach, and beef liver
- **B_6:** bananas, potatoes, fortified breakfast cereals, tuna, beef liver, and chickpeas

- **B₂ (riboflavin):** almonds, yogurt, dairy milk, oats, fortified breakfast cereals, and beef liver

Vitamin A

Vitamin A is essential for maintaining a healthy immune system and promoting good eye health due to its antioxidant properties. While it does not offer specific benefits during menopause, it can contribute to overall well-being and prevent certain diseases.

In the United States, vitamin A deficiency is uncommon, and it's important to note that excessive intake of supplemental vitamin A can lead to adverse effects. Therefore, it's recommended to consult a doctor before considering additional vitamin A supplementation.

Food sources rich in vitamin A include dried apricots, sweet potatoes, black-eyed peas, carrots, spinach, and beef liver.

Iron

Iron is commonly advised for younger women with extended or heavy menstrual cycles. However, it used to be believed that postmenopausal women could obtain sufficient iron from their diet alone. As a result, the daily recommended intake of iron decreases from 15 mg to 8 mg for postmenopausal women. However, the Women's Health Initiative (n.d), a large-scale study in 1991, uncovered that certain postmenopausal women may be susceptible to iron deficiency, commonly called anemia.

Fatigue and unexplained tiredness are prevalent symptoms of menopause, often associated with hormone fluctuations and the gradual decrease in menstrual cycles. As periods cease and hormone levels stabilize, many women experience a more consistent and stable energy level. However, if persistent tiredness and fatigue persevere beyond menopause, accompanied by symptoms such as lightheadedness, headaches, pale skin, and shortness of breath, it may indicate an iron deficiency rather than a solely hormone-related condition.

Both women and men need to exercise caution when considering iron supplementation. It's advisable to consult with a doctor and have your iron levels checked before starting any supplements. Excessive iron in the bloodstream can be just as harmful as having insufficient levels. In addition, iron tends to oxidize rapidly, and in its oxidized state it acts as a free radical, potentially causing damage to blood vessels, cells, and tissues in the body. Therefore, emphasizing iron-rich foods in your diet is a beneficial strategy for replenishing iron reserves.

Fluoride

While fluoride is an essential component in toothpaste and aids in improving bone density, it's not recommended as a treatment for menopausal bone loss. This is because fluoride is believed to increase the risk of fractures, so it's not explicitly used for addressing bone loss during menopause.

A study conducted in 2013 found that low-dose fluoride has no significant impact on skeletal health markers, and it's not a viable treatment option for osteoporosis. This supports the belief that fluoride is not practical for treating osteoporosis (Grey et al., 2013).

As more research expands our understanding of menopausal bone loss and effective treatment options, it's essential to consult health-care professionals who can provide personalized guidance and recommendations. In addition, they can help identify alternative approaches that demonstrate efficacy and safety for managing bone health during menopause.

To Summarize

The topic of supplements for menopause is multifaceted and dynamic, laying the foundation for our exploration of natural remedies in the next chapter. While we've delved into the effectiveness of supplements in managing menopause symptoms and discussed a range of options available to women, it's essential to approach them with caution and informed decision-making. Individual experiences may vary, and what works for one person may not work for another.

As we move forward, we'll keep discussing ways to manage menopause holistically. We will also investigate various natural treatments and lifestyle adjustments that may provide extra care and comfort during this significant phase. So, let's proceed with an open mind and embark on the journey of exploring natural solutions for menopause symptoms.

Chapter 5:

Natural Remedies for

Menopause

In this chapter, we delve into the world of herbal supplements for menopause. As women seek natural remedies to manage the symptoms of this transformative phase, herbal supplements have gained popularity as potential alternatives. As such, we will now explore a variety of herbal supplements commonly used to alleviate menopause symptoms.

From black cohosh to red clover, dong quai to evening primrose oil (EPO), we will discuss the benefits, potential side effects, and scientific evidence surrounding these herbal remedies. With a comprehensive understanding of these herbal supplements, you can make informed decisions about their use and discover natural options for alleviating discomfort during this critical stage of life.

Herbal Supplements

Women can use several herbal supplements to alleviate menopausal symptoms. However, the effectiveness of these supplements varies, and research suggests they may not be effective in relieving menopause symptoms ("Menopausal Symptoms: In Depth," 2017). In addition, it's crucial to remember that certain herbal supplements may have adverse reactions when taken with other medications and may not be suitable for everyone.

Before taking any vitamin or herbal supplements, it's essential to consult with your doctor or nurse. These supplements may interact with other medications and cause harmful effects, so it's crucial to seek professional advice. In addition, the FDA doesn't regulate supplements and medicines in the same way, so the safety and effectiveness of these supplements are not always well understood.

Ground Flaxseed

The effectiveness of flaxseed (also known as linseed) in alleviating hot flashes, as claimed by some individuals, is still uncertain based on mixed research findings. However, in a 3-month study involving 140 menopausal women, those who consumed flaxseeds reported notable improvements in multiple menopause symptoms and experienced an enhanced overall quality of life, according to their self-reports (Cetisli et al., 2015). Furthermore, an analysis of 11 studies concluded that flaxseeds were found to decrease the frequency and duration of hot flashes, but not significantly more than those who weren't taking flaxseeds (Dew & Williamson, 2013).

Nevertheless, the health benefits of flaxseeds are significant, mainly when consumed in ground form rather than as supplements. Consuming ground flaxseeds can provide your body with omega-3 fatty acids and lignans, linked to decreased cholesterol levels and a lower chance of developing breast cancer. Therefore, incorporating them into your diet can contribute to overall health, even if they do not provide relief from hot flashes.

Remember that flaxseeds contain phytoestrogens, compounds that can imitate the effects of estrogen in the body's tissues and cells. As a result, individuals undergoing uterine or breast cancer treatment should consult with their doctor before incorporating flaxseeds into their regimen.

Black Cohosh

Black cohosh is a natural remedy derived from the underground root and stems of the plant, which can be prepared as pills, capsules, tea, or liquid extracts. Throughout history, black cohosh has been used by Native Americans for various purposes, including managing fever, cough, and irregular menstruation. Additionally, European settlers incorporated black cohosh into their practices to promote female reproductive health.

In modern times, black cohosh has gained popularity as a potential remedy for menopausal symptoms, including hot flashes, night sweats, vaginal dryness, and irritability. However, two comprehensive reviews encompassing a substantial sample of over 8,000 perimenopausal, menopausal, and postmenopausal women concluded that the available evidence is inadequate to establish whether black cohosh holds superior efficacy compared with a placebo in alleviating menopause symptoms (Leach & Moore, 2012; Franco et al., 2016).

On the other hand, another study suggested that black cohosh can simulate the actions of essential neurotransmitters such as dopamine, serotonin, and norepinephrine, which can aid in alleviating depression and anxiety symptoms common in women going through menopause (Wuttke et al., 2014). However, the studies mentioned above noted that more research is needed to fully understand the herb's benefits.

Regardless, if you have a history of liver disease, it's not advisable to use black cohosh, as there have been reports of adverse reactions associated with contaminated supplements. Although adverse effects from black cohosh are infrequent, the National Institutes of Health states that the most commonly reported ones include mild symptoms such as nausea, stomach upset, and skin rashes ("Black Cohosh," 2020). Furthermore, they recommend selecting supplements with third-party purity testing for optimal safety and quality assurance.

Red Clover

The red clover is a flowering plant that falls under the legume family. It contains abundant isoflavones, which act similarly to estrogen and can potentially relieve symptoms related to decreased estrogen levels during menopause. Red clover is commonly used to manage or prevent menopausal symptoms such as hot flashes, night sweats, and bone loss. An analysis of 11 studies on menopausal women revealed that more women who received red clover reported a reduction in hot flashes compared with those who received a placebo (Ghazanfarpour et al., 2016).

Similarly, two earlier small-scale studies demonstrated that supplementation with red clover isoflavones may have the potential to decelerate bone loss in menopausal women when compared with a placebo (Clifton-Bligh et al., 2001; Atkinson et al., 2004).

While no severe adverse effects have been documented, it's essential to note that mild symptoms such as nausea and headache may occur when taking red clover. In addition, due to limited comprehensive safety information, it's recommended not to use red clover for more than 1 year. Finally, remember that red clover may not be appropriate for children, pregnant or breastfeeding women, or those with breast cancer or other hormone-sensitive cancers ("Red Clover," 2020).

Soy

Soybeans are abundant in isoflavones, which are similar to the hormone estrogen and can exert mild estrogenic effects within the body. The decline in estrogen production during menopause is often associated with various common symptoms.

Soy is believed to relieve these symptoms due to its estrogen-like properties. However, the existing evidence on this matter is inconclusive. While population studies suggest that a high soy intake is linked to a lower occurrence of hot flashes, large-scale clinical trials have shown limited significant benefits (Levis & Griebeler, 2010).

A thorough analysis of 95 studies focused on menopausal women has shown that taking soy isoflavone supplements may positively affect bone health and could potentially decrease the frequency and length of hot flashes. Nevertheless, it's essential to note that specific results cannot be guaranteed for every individual (Chen et al., 2019).

Soy-based foods like soybeans, tofu, and tempeh are considered safe and nutritious options for your diet. However, the long-term safety of high-soy isoflavone supplements is still uncertain. It's also worth noting that common side effects like diarrhea and stomach pain may occur. Therefore, it's recommended to consult with your health-care provider before incorporating soy isoflavone supplements into your daily routine.

Evening Primrose Oil

The evening primrose (*Oenothera biennis*) is a flowering plant that grows naturally in central and eastern North America. Its seeds extract EPO, which some women believe can relieve menopause symptoms like hot flashes. However, the findings from studies on the effectiveness of EPO are varied and inconclusive.

One study found that EPO did not show greater effectiveness than a placebo in reducing hot flashes (Farzaneh et al., 2013). By contrast, a more recent study indicated that EPO exhibited approximately 10% greater effectiveness in reducing the severity of hot flashes compared with a placebo (Johnson et al., 2019).

In another study involving pre- and postmenopausal women, the effects of a calcium supplement with a combined EPO, calcium, and omega-3 in preventing bone loss were compared. Both groups demonstrated preserved bone mineral density, but the EPO supplement did not show superior effectiveness to the calcium supplement (Johnson et al., 2019).

According to the National Center for Complementary and Integrative Health, most adults can safely use EPO for short-term purposes. It's generally well tolerated, and any reported side effects are usually mild, such as occasional stomach pain and nausea ("Evening Primrose Oil," n.d.). However, they further state that EPO may negatively interact with certain HIV drugs. Therefore, it's crucial to consult with your health-care provider before considering EPO, especially if you're taking other supplements or medications. Their guidance will help ensure your safety and avoid any potential complications.

Maca

For centuries, maca (*Lepidium meyenii*) has been used in traditional folk medicine to address various physical conditions, including anemia, infertility, hormonal imbalances, and specific symptoms associated with menopause, such as reduced libido, mood swings, and vaginal dryness (Lee et al., 2011).

The available evidence supporting the effectiveness of maca for menopause is limited in scope. Nevertheless, a few small-scale studies suggest that maca demonstrates a notable improvement over placebo in enhancing libido and alleviating psychological symptoms such as anxiety and depression (Brooks et al., 2008; Shin et al., 2010; Lee et al., 2011).

While no significant adverse effects have been reported regarding maca, limited safety data is available. It remains uncertain whether maca may interfere with medications, so it's advisable to consult with your health-care provider before incorporating it into your regimen.

It's essential to be cautious when obtaining maca, as its popularity has increased the risk of contamination and quality control issues during production. To ensure you're getting a safe product, purchasing maca from reputable sources is best.

Ginseng

Ginseng is widely recognized as one of the most popular herbal medicines globally. With a history of use spanning centuries in traditional Chinese medicine, it's believed to enhance immune function, promote heart health, and increase energy levels (Song et al., 2018).

Among the various types of ginseng available, Korean red ginseng has received the most attention concerning menopause. A comprehensive review of 10 studies indicated that Korean red ginseng might positively affect menopausal women, including boosting sex drive, improving mood, and enhancing overall well-being (Lee et al., 2016).

However, it's essential to note that the existing evidence for the effectiveness of Korean red ginseng in addressing menopausal symptoms is limited, and further research is necessary to establish its benefits conclusively.

In terms of safety, short-term use of Korean red ginseng is generally considered safe for most adults. However, it's vital to be aware of potential side effects, including skin rash, diarrhea, dizziness, difficulty sleeping, and headache. Additionally, individuals with diabetes should exercise caution as Korean red ginseng may interfere with blood sugar control. Therefore, talking to your health-care provider before using Korean red ginseng is recommended, particularly if you have diabetes or are taking medications that may interact with it (Song et al., 2018; "Asian ginseng," 2020).

Ginseng can interact adversely with certain medications for blood pressure, cholesterol, and blood-thinning purposes. Therefore, it's crucial to seek advice from your health-care provider before considering using ginseng, mainly if you take any of these medications.

Chasteberry

Chasteberry, scientifically known as *Vitex agnus-castus*, is an herbal remedy that originates from Asia and the Mediterranean regions. It has a history of traditional use in addressing conditions such as infertility, menstrual disorders, and symptoms associated with menopause and premenstrual syndrome (PMS).

The research on the effectiveness of chasteberry in alleviating menopause symptoms is inconclusive, much like other herbal remedies. For example, a study involving 92 women given either a placebo or a combination of chasteberry and St. John's wort did not find any significant differences in menopause symptoms between the two groups (van Die et al., 2009). On the other hand, in another study involving 52 women who took chasteberry, significant reductions in anxiety and hot flashes were observed. However, there were no notable changes in depression or sexual dysfunction reported (Naseri et al., 2019).

Chasteberry is generally considered safe, although mild side effects such as digestive discomfort, headache, itchy skin, and nausea may occur. It's important to note that if you're taking antipsychotic medications or drugs, it's not recommended to try chasteberry.

Valerian

Valerian (*Valeriana officinalis*) is a flowering plant known for its calming and relaxation-inducing properties, with its roots commonly used in various herbal medicine traditions. Valerian, often called "nature's Valium," can be used to treat menopause symptoms such as insomnia and hot flashes. Although there is a lack of substantial evidence supporting its effectiveness, preliminary findings are encouraging.

In a study involving 68 menopausal women, valerian supplements were notably more effective in reducing the subjective severity of hot flashes than a placebo (Mirabi & Mojab, 2013). Similarly, a study involving 60 menopausal women reported similar positive outcomes (Jenabi et al., 2017). Another study with 100 menopausal women showed that a combination of lemon balm and valerian improved their sleep quality significantly compared with those who took a placebo (Taavoni et al., 2013).

Valerian is generally considered safe, although it may cause mild side effects, including digestive upset, headaches, drowsiness, and dizziness. If you're taking medications for anxiety, pain, or sleep, it's not recommended to take valerian, as it may have a compounding effect. Additionally, it may interact negatively with supplements such as St. John's wort, melatonin, and kava. Therefore, it's essential to consult with your health-care provider before combining valerian with any medications or supplements.

Dong Quai

Dong quai (*Angelica sinensis*), commonly referred to as female ginseng, is an herb native to Asia and closely related to celery, carrot, and parsley. It thrives in cooler regions, mainly China, Korea, and Japan. In traditional Chinese medicine, dong quai is often used to promote women's health and alleviate symptoms of PMS and menopause.

Despite being widely used, limited scientific research is available to substantiate dong quai's effectiveness for menopause symptoms. For example, a study involving 71 women comparing the effects of dong quai versus placebo did not find any significant differences in the alleviation of vaginal dryness or reduction of hot flashes (Geller & Studee, 2005).

However, in another study where dong quai was combined with other herbs like chamomile, black cohosh, and red clover, it was found to significantly reduce the frequency and intensity of hot flashes and night sweats (Johnson et al., 2019). Ultimately, further research is required to understand the effectiveness of dong quai for menopause symptoms fully.

Dong quai is generally considered safe for most adults, although it's important to note that it may increase sensitivity to sunlight. Additionally, dong quai may have a blood-thinning effect, so individuals taking blood thinners should avoid it.

Wild Yam

Many practitioners of alternative medicine suggest using wild yam as a natural substitute for estrogen replacement therapy to help relieve menopause symptoms. The underlying belief is that wild yam has the potential to enhance or stabilize estrogen levels in the body, thus providing relief from various symptoms associated with menopause.

Nevertheless, the available evidence to support these assertions is minimal. For example, one of the few studies on this subject examined the effects of a wild yam cream applied by 23 women over a 3-month duration, and found no discernible changes in their menopausal symptoms (Komesaroff et al., 2001).

Flaxseed Oil and Vitamin E

To address vaginal dryness and improve lubrication, individuals can apply topical flaxseed or vitamin E oil to the vaginal area. These natural remedies are believed to nourish and moisturize the vaginal tissues, relieving discomfort.

Additionally, research indicates that using vitamin E suppositories may effectively alleviate symptoms of vaginal atrophy, a condition characterized by thinning, inflammation, and dryness of the vaginal walls (Emamverdikhan et al., 2016). However, consulting with a health-care professional before initiating any new treatment is essential to ensure its appropriateness and safety for individual circumstances.

To Summarize

Exploring natural remedies for menopause can offer individuals a range of potential benefits in managing their symptoms. However, while many natural remedies have shown promising results and have been used traditionally for centuries, it's crucial to consider the evidence supporting their effectiveness and potential risks. Therefore, it's recommended to consult with health-care professionals to understand the benefits and risks of specific natural remedies.

In the upcoming chapter, we'll delve into the intricate relationship between menopause and mental health, examining the various challenges faced and strategies for fostering emotional resilience. Join us as we navigate the terrain of mental health during menopause, offering insights and guidance to help you navigate this transformative journey with grace and empowerment.

Chapter 6:

Mental Health and

Menopause

Navigating the complexities of menopause involves not only physical changes but also significant impacts on mental health and emotional well-being. In this chapter, we will explore the intricate relationship between menopause and mental health, shedding light on the various psychological aspects that women may encounter during this transformative phase. From mood swings to anxiety and depression, we will delve into the common mental health challenges experienced by menopausal women and provide insights into strategies for managing and promoting mental well-being.

The Impact of Menopause on Mental Health

Decreasing estrogen levels can make you feel like you're in a perpetual state of PMS. As discussed in Chapter 1, let's briefly revisit some of the emotional changes that you may experience during perimenopause or menopause:

- unexplained physical pain or discomfort

- changes in appetite, resulting in alterations to your eating habits

- disturbed sleep patterns, either sleeping too little or too much

- decreased energy levels and feelings of fatigue

- memory lapses or forgetfulness

- difficulties concentrating or making decisions

- loss of interest in activities that previously brought you joy

- sensations of guilt or worthlessness

- feelings of anxiety, restlessness, or agitation

- increased irritability, frustration, or episodes of angry outbursts

Experiencing crankiness and sadness may be associated with menopause, but it's essential to consider other factors that could be contributing to these emotions. Discussing your feelings with your doctor to exclude any underlying medical or psychiatric conditions is recommended.

The mental health symptoms encountered during menopause can stem from various causes, indicating that hormonal changes alone may not be the sole contributor. Factors such as significant life stressors experienced during one's 40s and 50s can also play a role in exacerbating symptoms like depression. In addition, balancing responsibilities like caring for aging parents, raising children, and coping with work-related stress can all contribute to the complex interplay of mental well-being during this transformative phase.

Furthermore, specific physical manifestations of menopause can directly influence mental health. For example, menopause is not the only time when women experience symptoms such as hot flashes, disrupted sleep patterns, diminished energy levels, and weight fluctuations. Still, they can also significantly impact overall quality of life, including mental well-being. Moreover, specific physical indicators of menopause, such as hot flashes, can resemble symptoms of anxiety and panic attacks.

Contributing Factors

Specific individuals may exhibit a heightened susceptibility to the mental health impacts of menopause compared with others. One significant determinant is a previous history of mental health difficulties. For instance, as stated by the North American Menopause Society, the most influential contributing factor to the onset of depression during menopause is a personal background of mental health challenges or periods of depressive mood experienced earlier in life ("Depression & Menopause," n.d.).

Several factors can contribute to increased mental health challenges during menopause. These include:

- **Intense physical discomfort:** The physical side effects of menopause, particularly hot flashes, can cause significant discomfort and disrupt daily life. These discomforts can impact mental well-being.

- **Lack of social and emotional support:** Menopause can be challenging, and a robust support system is crucial. The absence of adequate social and emotional support can exacerbate mental health issues during this phase.

- **Life changes and challenges:** Menopause often coincides with significant changes, such as children leaving the nest or caring for aging parents. Dealing with these transitions alongside the hormonal changes of menopause can contribute to heightened mental health challenges.

- **Unhealthy lifestyle behaviors:** Neglecting positive health behaviors, such as maintaining a healthy diet or engaging in regular exercise, can negatively impact both physical and mental well-being during menopause.

- **Sleep disturbances:** Sleep disruptions are expected during menopause, and a consistent lack of sleep can affect mental health. The combination of hormonal changes and other menopausal symptoms can make it difficult to get restful sleep, leading to increased mental health challenges.

- **Emergence of other health issues:** Menopause can coincide with the onset of other health conditions, such as thyroid issues, which can further disrupt hormonal balance and contribute to mental health issues. It's vital to address these underlying health concerns during menopause to mitigate their impact on mental well-being.

Treating Menopause-Related Mental Health Issues

Therapy

Biofeedback and Relaxation Training

To reduce the occurrence of hot flashes and ease the psychological symptoms linked to perimenopause, relaxation techniques like progressive muscle relaxation can be helpful (Johnson et al., 2019). However, further research is needed to establish their effectiveness conclusively.

Biofeedback techniques involve monitoring and controlling physiological responses to improve overall self-regulation. When combined with relaxation training, such as progressive muscle relaxation, individuals can learn to recognize and manage their body's reactions to stress, potentially reducing the frequency and intensity of hot flashes. These techniques also promote a sense of calmness and relaxation, which can alleviate psychological symptoms commonly associated with perimenopause.

Cognitive Behavioral Therapy

According to one article, certain studies have indicated that cognitive behavioral therapy (CBT) may aid in reducing mild depression and the frequency of hot flashes (Johnson et al., 2019). CBT is a therapeutic approach that identifies and modifies negative thought patterns and behaviors. By addressing the underlying causes of mild depression and hot flashes, CBT empowers individuals to develop effective coping strategies which promote positive changes in their mental and emotional well-being.

Hypnosis

One study revealed that hypnosis was comparable in effectiveness to venlafaxine, a commonly prescribed medication for reducing hot flashes (Barton et al., 2017).

This suggests that hypnosis can be a viable alternative treatment.

In addition to being an alternative to medication, hypnosis offers a non-invasive approach that can be tailored to an individual's specific needs. Hypnosis uses the power of the mind to induce relaxation and positive mental states. This can be beneficial in reducing hot flashes and promoting overall well-being.

Mindfulness-Based Stress Reduction

Mindfulness-based stress reduction (MBSR) incorporates a range of practices, including various exercises like yoga and meditation, to enhance well-being and lower stress levels. For example, the National Institute on Aging suggests that yoga, tai chi, and mindfulness meditation can help alleviate hot flashes ("Hot Flashes: What Can I Do?," 2021).

Additionally, as indicated by one study, MBSR has been deemed safe and has shown potential benefits, including improved sleep quality, anxiety reduction, and stress reduction (Johnson et al., 2019). However, it's essential to acknowledge that further research is needed to fully understand the impact of these practices on vasomotor symptoms, such as hot flashes and night sweats.

Talk Therapy

The experience of feeling isolated can hinder your inclination to share your feelings and experiences with friends or family members. However, seeking the support of a trained therapist can provide a more conducive space to discuss and navigate the challenges you're facing. In addition, speaking with a therapist can offer a sense of ease and comfort, allowing you to address and cope with the difficulties you're encountering openly.

Medications

Hormone Replacement Therapy

We discussed HRT at length in Chapter 3, but it's essential to mention it again in the context of mental health. The use of synthetic hormones can be beneficial in addressing specific mental health challenges that occur during menopause. According to the North American Menopause Society, estrogen, in particular, can improve mood and protect against depression ("Depression & Menopause," n.d.). HRT can be used as a standalone treatment or in combination with antidepressant medications.

Low-Dose Estrogen Replacement Therapy

Estrogen replacement therapy, prescribed by your doctor, can be administered through oral pills or skin patches. This therapy may alleviate both the physical and emotional symptoms associated with menopause.

Antidepressants

The North American Menopause Society suggests using SSRIs to address depression and anxiety associated with menopause ("Depression & Menopause," n.d.). However, it's essential to note that SSRIs may sometimes lead to sexual side effects like reduced desire and difficulty reaching orgasm. If you experience sexual side effects from SSRIs, it's suggested to explore other options like bupropion or duloxetine that have fewer of these effects. Therefore, it's essential to consult with your health-care provider to determine the most suitable antidepressant option for you.

Aromatherapy Massage

Aromatherapy has emerged as a different approach to address the psychological symptoms of perimenopause. In a study involving 90 participants, the combination of aromatherapy and massage demonstrated notable benefits in reducing psychological symptoms commonly associated with this transitional phase (Darsareh et al., 2012).

By incorporating aromatic plant extracts, such as essential oils, along with the therapeutic touch of massage, individuals may experience improved emotional well-being and relief from symptoms like stress, anxiety, and mood fluctuations. However, further research is needed to explore aromatherapy's specific mechanisms and potential long-term effects in managing perimenopausal symptoms.

Dealing With Menopause-Related Mental Health Issues

Prioritize Self-Care

During the midlife phase, we often find ourselves juggling various responsibilities, such as guiding our children toward independence, navigating an empty nest, and attending to the needs of aging parents. All the while, we are typically maintaining our jobs and managing household duties. Amid this busyness, carving out time for self-care can be challenging. However, it's crucial to prioritize self-care as it can significantly benefit our mental well-being.

Make Lifestyle Changes

Incorporating specific lifestyle adjustments can contribute to mitigating the physical and psychological effects of menopause. These adjustments encompass adopting a nourishing, well-rounded diet, engaging in regular physical activity, and emphasizing sufficient sleep, all of which will be discussed in the following chapter.

To Summarize

The process of menopause is affected by hormonal changes that can lead to distressing physical symptoms like hot flashes and disruptions in sleep patterns. Additionally, individuals often encounter heightened mood swings and an increased likelihood of experiencing symptoms related to depression or anxiety. Fortunately, assistance is available for those facing the mental health implications of menopause. Whether you seek guidance from your gynecologist or consult a trained mental health professional, support is accessible to help improve your well-being.

We now shift our focus to beneficial lifestyle changes in Chapter 6. This chapter will delve into practical strategies that can enhance your physical and emotional well-being during the menopausal transition. From adopting a nutritious diet and engaging in regular exercise to managing stress and prioritizing self-care, we will explore the power of lifestyle modifications in navigating this phase of life.

Chapter 7:

Beneficial Lifestyle

Changes

It's time to discuss practical strategies to empower you during this transformative phase. This chapter will delve into the significance of adopting a nutritious diet, engaging in regular exercise, managing stress, and prioritizing self-care.

By embracing these lifestyle modifications, you can enhance your physical and emotional well-being and navigate the menopausal transition with grace and vitality. This chapter will provide practical tips, expert advice, and inspiration to help you integrate these strategies into your daily life, empowering you to embrace this transformative phase with confidence and resilience.

Eat Foods Rich in Phytoestrogen, Calcium, and Iron

Maintaining a healthy diet during menopause is crucial for overall well-being and managing various symptoms. As hormonal changes occur, it becomes essential to prioritize nutrient-rich foods that provide the necessary vitamins, minerals, and antioxidants. It's critical for women who experience menopause to eat lots of phytoestrogen-rich foods, calcium-rich foods, and iron-rich foods.

Phytoestrogen-Rich Foods

A systematic review indicated that phytoestrogens show promise in reducing the frequency of hot flashes (Chen et al., 2014). In addition, another article stated that incorporating phytoestrogens into the diet may decrease the likelihood of experiencing symptoms during perimenopause (Rietjens et al., 2016). Nevertheless, the article also mentioned that the available data on phytoestrogens is insufficient and highlights potential health risks associated with their consumption.

Therefore, if an individual chooses to incorporate foods rich in phytoestrogens into their diet, it's advisable to do so in moderation and as part of a well-balanced overall dietary approach. This means that phytoestrogen-rich foods should not be relied upon as the sole solution for managing menopause symptoms or as a replacement for medical advice or treatment.

Some foods that are high in phytoestrogens include:

- **Sesame seeds:** Sesame seeds are tiny seeds used widely in cooking and baking. They are rich in lignans, which have estrogenic properties. Sesame seeds can be sprinkled on salads and stir-fries or used to make tahini, a popular ingredient in Middle Eastern cuisine.

- **Edamame beans:** Edamame beans are young soybeans harvested before they fully mature. They are often boiled or steamed, served as a nutritious snack, or added to salads, stir-fries, or soups. Edamame beans are an excellent source of isoflavones and offer a range of health benefits.

- **Soy protein:** Soy protein is derived from soybeans and is a versatile plant-based protein source. Soybeans contain isoflavones, which act as phytoestrogens in the body. Consuming soy protein may help alleviate menopausal symptoms such as hot flashes and promote heart health.

- **Tofu:** Tofu, or bean curd, is made from soy milk. It's a versatile food used in various savory and sweet dishes. Tofu is an excellent source of isoflavones and provides essential nutrients such as protein, calcium, and iron.

- **Tempeh:** Tempeh is a fermented soybean product originating from Indonesia. It's a good source of isoflavones, including genistein and daidzein. Tempeh is known for its nutty flavor and firm texture, making it a popular ingredient in vegetarian and vegan dishes.

- **Flaxseed:** Flaxseed is a tiny seed high in lignans, a type of phytoestrogen. Lignans have been studied for their potential estrogenic effects and their role in promoting hormone balance. Flaxseed can be ground and added to various dishes, such as smoothies, cereals, or baked goods.

- **Miso:** Miso is a traditional Japanese seasoning made from fermented soybeans, grains, and salt. It's rich in phytoestrogens and offers a range of health benefits. Miso soup, a famous Japanese dish, is a common way to incorporate miso into the diet.

- **Broccoli:** Broccoli is a cruciferous vegetable that contains a compound called indole-3-carbinol. This compound may have estrogen-modulating effects and has been studied for its potential to reduce the risk of certain cancers, including breast and cervical cancer.

Calcium-Rich Foods and Vitamin D

During the perimenopausal phase, individuals may experience a decrease in bone density, making it crucial to prioritize bone health. Calcium and vitamin D are essential nutrients that help maintain strong bones, particularly in postmenopausal individuals.

There are various dairy options available that are rich in calcium, including:

- **Milk:** Milk is a classic source of calcium. Reduce your calorie intake while still getting the calcium benefits of milk by choosing low-fat or skim varieties.

- **Cheese:** Different types of cheese, such as cottage cheese, mozzarella, and cheddar, provide significant amounts of calcium to support bone health.

- **Yogurt:** Yogurt is a delicious and convenient source of calcium. Opt for low-fat or Greek yogurt for a healthy choice.

For those who prefer non-dairy alternatives, there are also options to consider:

- **Chia seeds:** While not a dairy product, chia seeds are a great plant-based source of calcium. Sprinkle them on yogurt, add them to smoothies, or use them as an ingredient in baking to boost your calcium intake.

- **Tofu:** Tofu is a versatile plant-based protein source that also contains calcium. Add tofu to stir-fries, salads, or other dishes to increase calcium intake.

- **Soy milk:** Fortified soy milk is a popular non-dairy option with calcium content similar to cow's milk. It can be enjoyed as a beverage or used in various recipes.

By including these calcium-rich foods in your diet, whether from dairy or non-dairy sources, you can contribute to maintaining healthy bones. Additionally, it's vital to ensure adequate vitamin D intake, as it supports the absorption and use of calcium in the body. You can obtain vitamin D from a variety of food sources. Some examples include:

- **Milk:** Cow's milk is often fortified with vitamin D, making it a good source of this essential nutrient. Enjoying a glass of milk can give you a vitamin D dose.

- **Soy milk:** Fortified soy milk is another option for obtaining vitamin D. Check the label to ensure it's fortified with vitamin D.

- **Cheddar cheese:** Cheddar cheese is a delicious dairy product that can contribute to your vitamin D intake. Enjoy it in moderation as part of a balanced diet.

- **Mushrooms:** Certain mushrooms, such as shiitake and maitake, naturally contain vitamin D. Including them in your meals can be a tasty way to boost your vitamin D levels.

- **Lentils:** While less rich in vitamin D than animal-based sources, lentils are a plant-based option that contains small amounts of this nutrient. Including lentils in your meals adds variety and nutritional value.

- **Fortified breakfast cereals:** Some breakfast cereals are fortified with vitamin D, providing a convenient way to incorporate this nutrient into your morning routine. Look for cereals that specifically mention vitamin D fortification on the label.

- **Fish:** Fatty fish like salmon, trout, and sardines are excellent sources of vitamin D. Including these fish in your diet can contribute to your vitamin D intake.

Incorporating these vitamin-D-rich foods into your diet can help support your overall vitamin D levels. However, it's important to note that sunlight exposure is a primary source of vitamin D for most people.

Consult a health-care professional or registered dietitian for personalized guidance on meeting your calcium and vitamin D needs during menopause.

Iron-Rich Foods

Including iron-rich foods in your diet can help alleviate symptoms such as hot flashes, heart palpitations, insomnia, and irritability. Various foods are excellent sources of iron, including:

- **Kidney beans:** Kidney beans are a legume that is rich in iron and can be incorporated into various dishes.

- **Dark chocolate:** Indulging in dark chocolate can offer a delicious way to increase your iron levels.

- **Tomatoes:** Tomatoes are a versatile fruit that contains iron and can be used in salads or sauces, or enjoyed on their own.

- **Cashew nuts:** Snacking on cashew nuts can provide you with iron while also offering a satisfying crunch.

- **Green vegetables:** Broccoli, spinach, kale, asparagus, and parsley are all examples of green vegetables that are packed with iron and can be included in your meals to enhance iron intake.

- **Fortified breakfast cereals:** Look for breakfast cereals that are fortified with iron to boost your iron intake.

- **White beans:** White beans, also known as cannellini beans, are another nutritious legume that provides a good amount of iron.

Including these iron-rich foods in your diet may help alleviate the mentioned symptoms. However, it's essential to maintain a balanced diet and consult with a health-care professional or registered dietitian to ensure you meet your specific nutritional needs.

Avoid Trigger Foods

Specific foods that may act as triggers can influence mood changes, night sweats, and hot flashes. These triggers might have a more substantial effect when consumed during nighttime.

Frequently reported triggers include caffeine, alcohol, and foods high in sugar or spiciness. To better understand how certain foods impact your menopause symptoms, it can be helpful to maintain a symptom diary. By keeping track of your experiences, you can identify any patterns or associations between certain foods and your symptoms. If you notice that particular foods consistently trigger your menopause symptoms, you may consider reducing your intake or eliminating them from your diet entirely. This personalized approach can help you manage and alleviate the effects of these triggers on your well-being.

Eat Plenty of Fruits and Vegetables

Consuming a diet abundant in fruits and vegetables can contribute to the prevention of various symptoms associated with menopause. Fruits and vegetables are naturally low in calories and high in dietary fiber, making them beneficial for weight loss and weight management goals. In addition, their high fiber content can promote satiety and reduce overall calorie intake.

Furthermore, including fruits and vegetables in your diet has been linked to a decreased risk of several diseases, including heart disease (Wang et al., 2014). Therefore, after menopause, it's crucial to prioritize heart health as the risk of heart disease tends to rise during this phase of life. This increase in risk could be attributed to various factors, including age, weight gain, and potentially decreased estrogen levels.

Moreover, incorporating ample amounts of fruits and vegetables into your diet may also contribute to preventing bone loss. An observational study involving 3,236 women aged 50–59 discovered that diets rich in fruits and vegetables were associated with reduced bone breakdown, indicating a potential protective effect on bone health (Hardcastle et al., 2010).

Eat Protein-Rich Foods

Incorporating protein into your meals consistently throughout the day can be beneficial in mitigating age-related loss of lean muscle mass. In addition, distributing protein intake evenly across meals can help slow down the muscle loss commonly associated with aging.

Beyond its muscle-preserving effects, a high-protein diet can also aid in weight loss by promoting satiety and boosting calorie expenditure. Excellent protein sources include nuts, legumes, eggs, fish, meat, and dairy products. Prioritizing protein-rich foods can support muscle maintenance and potentially enhance your weight-management efforts.

Eat Less Processed Food and Refined Sugar

Consuming a diet predominantly composed of refined carbohydrates and added sugars can lead to rapid fluctuations in blood sugar levels, resulting in fatigue and irritability. These fluctuations in blood sugar levels can potentially exacerbate the physical and mental symptoms associated with menopause. Interestingly, a study has revealed that diets rich in refined carbs may heighten the risk of depression among postmenopausal women (Gangwisch et al., 2015).

The consumption of diets high in processed foods can negatively impact bone health, particularly when these foods replace the essential nutrients obtained from a well-balanced daily diet. For example, an extensive observational study revealed that women aged 50–59 who consumed diets rich in processed and snack foods displayed lower bone quality (Aucott et al., 2010).

Don't Skip Meals

Establishing a routine of regular meals can be crucial during the menopausal phase. Irregular eating patterns can exacerbate specific menopausal symptoms and hinder effective weight management. A study conducted over a year focusing on weight management in postmenopausal women revealed that skipping meals was linked to a 4.3% reduction in weight loss (Kong et al., 2012). This underscores the significance of maintaining consistent meal habits to support overall well-being and achieve weight-related goals during menopause.

Stay Hydrated

Several researchers recommend a daily intake of at least 8–12 glasses of water for optimal health (Chopra et al., 2019). Not only can drinking enough water daily contribute to reducing hot flashes, but since individuals may be more susceptible to urinary tract infections during perimenopause, maintaining proper hydration by drinking ample water can assist in preventing recurring infections. Staying hydrated can also effectively alleviate bloating, commonly associated with hormonal changes during menopause.

Furthermore, water can play a significant role in weight management. By keeping you adequately hydrated, it can contribute to preventing weight gain and supporting weight loss efforts. Water can make you feel fuller, reducing the likelihood of overeating, and it can also help slightly boost your metabolism. By incorporating sufficient water intake into your daily routine, you can promote a healthy weight and support your overall well-being during the menopausal transition.

Consuming two cups of water approximately 30 minutes before a meal has been associated with a potential reduction in calorie intake during the meal, with studies suggesting a decrease of around 13% in calories consumed (Davy et al., 2008). By drinking water before a meal, you may experience a greater feeling of fullness, leading to a natural reduction in food intake. This simple practice can be a helpful strategy for managing calorie intake and supporting weight management goals.

Manage Your Weight

Hormonal changes, muscle loss, disrupted sleep, and insulin resistance are expected consequences of menopause that can contribute to an increased risk of weight gain. In addition, the accumulation of excessive body fat, particularly in the abdominal area, raises the likelihood of developing various health conditions, including heart disease and diabetes.

Moreover, body weight has the potential to impact the experience of menopausal symptoms. For example, according to a study conducted on 17,473 postmenopausal women, those who achieved a weight loss of at least 10 pounds (4.5 kg) or 10% of their body weight within one year had a higher likelihood of experiencing a resolution of hot flashes and night sweats (Kroenke et al., 2012).

Three diet plans have proven effective in losing weight during menopause and after: a vegetarian or vegan diet, a Mediterranean diet, and a low-carb diet.

Vegetarian/Vegan Diet

A vegetarian diet is a dietary approach that excludes the consumption of meat, poultry, seafood, and sometimes other animal-derived products. On the other hand, a vegan diet is a more strict form of vegetarianism that avoids all animal-derived products, including meat, poultry, seafood, eggs, dairy, honey, and other animal ingredients. The core components of both diets include:

- **Fruits and vegetables:** These are essential sources of vitamins, minerals, fiber, and antioxidants. They form the foundation of vegan and vegetarian diets, providing a wide range of nutrients.

- **Grains and legumes:** Whole grains (such as quinoa, brown rice, and oats) and legumes (such as beans, lentils, and chickpeas) are excellent sources of complex carbohydrates, protein, and fiber. They contribute to satiety and provide essential nutrients.

- **Nuts and seeds:** These are nutrient-dense foods that offer healthy fats, protein, fiber, vitamins, and minerals. They can be included as snacks or incorporated into meals, adding flavor, texture, and nutritional benefits.

- **Plant-based protein sources:** Tofu, tempeh, seitan, and plant-based protein powders are common alternatives to animal-based proteins. They provide essential amino acids and can be used in various recipes.

Both vegan and vegetarian diets have demonstrated potential for weight loss. For example, research conducted on postmenopausal women revealed noteworthy weight reduction and health improvements in those following a vegan diet (Barnard et al., 2005; Turner-McGrievy et al., 2012). Additionally, one survey showed that individuals following a vegan diet during perimenopause reported experiencing less severe vasomotor symptoms, including hot flashes, and exhibited fewer physical symptoms than those following an omnivorous diet (Beezhold et al., 2018). Nonetheless, a flexible vegetarian approach incorporating dairy and eggs has also demonstrated positive outcomes among older women (Mahon et al., 2007).

Mediterranean Diet

The Mediterranean diet is a dietary pattern inspired by the traditional eating habits of countries bordering the Mediterranean Sea, such as Greece, Italy, Spain, and France. It emphasizes consuming whole, minimally processed foods commonly found in the Mediterranean region. Some key features of the diet include:

- **Abundant plant-based foods:** The diet is rich in fruits, vegetables, legumes, whole grains, nuts, and seeds. These foods provide a wide array of vitamins, minerals, antioxidants, and fiber.

- **Healthy fats:** The Mediterranean diet encourages the consumption of healthy fats, primarily in olive oil as the primary source of added fat. Other sources of healthy fats include nuts, seeds, and avocados.

- **Moderate consumption of dairy and fish:** Dairy products, particularly fermented options like yogurt and cheese, are consumed in moderation. Fish and seafood, rich in omega-3 fatty acids, are also part of the diet, typically consumed a few times weekly.

- **Little red meat and processed foods:** Red meat is consumed sparingly in the Mediterranean diet, focusing on leaner protein sources like poultry and legumes. Processed foods, refined grains, and added sugars are also limited.

- **Herbs and spices:** The diet incorporates a variety of herbs and spices to enhance flavor, reducing the need for excessive salt and unhealthy seasonings.

While the Mediterranean diet is widely recognized for its health benefits and ability to lower the risk of heart disease, research indicates that it can also promote weight loss (Mancini et al., 2016; Sayón-Orea et al., 2015). It's important to note that most studies on the Mediterranean diet have examined its effects on men and women rather than focusing specifically on perimenopausal or postmenopausal women. However, one study on individuals aged 55 years and older, including both men and women, found that following a Mediterranean diet significantly reduced abdominal fat (Babio et al., 2014).

Low Carb Diet

A low-carb diet is a dietary approach that reduces the consumption of carbohydrates, particularly those high in refined sugars and starches. The main principle of a low-carb diet is to limit the intake of foods such as bread, pasta, rice, potatoes, and candy.

Instead, a low-carb diet emphasizes foods high in protein, healthy fats, and non-starchy vegetables. Everyday food choices on a low-carb diet include:

- **Protein sources:** Lean meats (e.g., chicken and turkey), fish, eggs, and dairy products (e.g., Greek yogurt, cheese).

- **Healthy fats:** Avocados, nuts and seeds (e.g., almonds, walnuts, chia seeds), olive oil, coconut oil, and fatty fish (e.g., salmon, mackerel).
- **Non-starchy vegetables:** Leafy greens (e.g., spinach, kale, lettuce), broccoli, cauliflower, bell peppers, zucchini, and asparagus.

Numerous studies have consistently demonstrated the effectiveness of low-carb diets for weight loss and their ability to specifically target and reduce abdominal fat (Goss et al., 2014; Johnston et al., 2014; Gower & Goss, 2014). Nevertheless, while perimenopausal and postmenopausal women have been participants in various low-carb studies, limited research focuses explicitly on this population.

However, a notable study examining postmenopausal women revealed significant weight loss results within 6 months. The participants following a low-carb diet achieved a remarkable reduction of 21.8 pounds, 27.5% of body fat, and 3.5 inches from their waists (Thompson et al., 2015).

Furthermore, achieving weight loss does not necessarily require a deficient intake of carbohydrates. An additional study compared the effects of a paleo diet, which provided approximately 30% of calories from carbs, versus a low-fat diet, where 55–60% of calories came from carbs. The results showed that after 2 years, the paleo diet led to a more significant reduction in abdominal fat and overall weight than the low-fat diet (Mellberg et al., 2014).

Regardless of your diet, be sure to incorporate foods high in phytoestrogen, calcium, vitamin D, and iron. Additionally, no weight-loss regimen will be complete without exercise.

Exercise Regularly

Exercise can be beneficial for relieving menopause symptoms such as hot flashes, insomnia, mood changes, and weight gain. One study revealed that individuals who engaged in moderate to high levels of physical activity experienced milder symptoms than inactive individuals (Dąbrowska-Galas et al., 2019).

Another study discovered that although 12 weeks of moderate exercise did not directly alleviate vasomotor symptoms, it did show potential benefits by improving symptoms of depression, insomnia, and sleep quality (Sternfeld et al., 2013). According to a suggested guideline in a research article, individuals are encouraged to engage in 150 minutes of moderate-intensity physical activity per week (Chopra et al., 2019).

Maintaining an active lifestyle and incorporating various forms of exercise into your routine can significantly contribute to alleviating menopause symptoms and promoting overall well-being. Whether engaging in aerobic activities like walking or cycling, strength training exercises, yoga, tai chi, or Pilates, each exercise offers unique benefits.

Remember to consult your health-care provider before starting any new exercise program, especially if you have underlying health conditions. By embracing regular physical activity and prioritizing it in your life, you can enhance your physical and mental health during the menopausal transition, helping you navigate this transformative stage with greater comfort and vitality.

Strength Training

Given the increased risk of osteoporosis after menopause, it becomes crucial to prioritize strength training. These exercises are vital in building bone density and muscle strength while aiding in fat burning and boosting metabolism.

When exercising at home, consider using dumbbells and resistance tubing. In addition, you can opt for weight machines or free weights if you prefer the gym setting. Start with a weight level that challenges your muscles within 12 repetitions and gradually progress.

Cardio

According to the Centers for Disease Control and Prevention (CDC), individuals who are new to exercise should begin with 10 minutes of light activity and gradually increase the intensity as their fitness level improves ("How Much Physical Activity Do Adults Need?" 2022). Engaging in aerobic activities that involve large muscle groups and elevate your heart rate is highly beneficial. The possibilities for cardiovascular exercises are endless, as nearly any physical activity, such as walking, jogging, cycling, and swimming, can be considered.

Walking

Walking is a simple yet effective exercise that can easily be incorporated into your daily routine. It offers numerous benefits for your overall health and well-being. Not only does walking improve cardiovascular health and strengthen bones, but it also helps maintain a healthy weight. Additionally, walking positively impacts mental well-being by reducing stress levels and improving mood. Finally, taking regular walks can provide a refreshing break, allowing you to clear your mind and enjoy the beauty of nature.

Jogging

Jogging is a higher-intensity aerobic exercise that benefits your body and mind. Engaging in regular jogging sessions can significantly enhance your cardiovascular fitness and increase bone density, which is particularly important during menopause. Jogging also helps burn calories, improve muscle tone, and boost stamina. Moreover, this exercise releases endorphins, the feel-good hormones which can alleviate mood swings and reduce symptoms of anxiety and depression. It's time to put on your running shoes and experience the exhilaration of jogging as you improve your physical and mental well-being.

Cycling

Cycling is a low-impact exercise that offers fantastic cardiovascular benefits while being gentle on your joints. Whether you prefer outdoor cycling or using a stationary bike, this activity can significantly improve your overall fitness. Cycling strengthens the lower-body muscles, including the legs and buttocks, while helping to maintain joint flexibility. It's also a fantastic way to explore the outdoors, reduce stress, and improve mental clarity. Feel the wind in your hair and enjoy the refreshing cycling experience as you care for your physical and psychological health.

Swimming

Swimming is a fantastic full-body workout that provides both physical and mental benefits. As a low-impact exercise, swimming is gentle on the joints, making it an ideal choice for menopausal women. It improves cardiovascular health, tones muscles throughout the body, and enhances flexibility. One of the unique advantages of swimming during menopause is its ability to cool the body and alleviate hot flashes. Additionally, swimming promotes relaxation and can improve sleep quality, allowing you to experience a more profound sense of rejuvenation and well-being.

Boxing

Boxing is an exhilarating and empowering exercise with many physical and mental benefits. Engaging in boxing workouts helps strengthen the heart muscles, lower the risk of heart disease, and combat menopause-related weight gain. It also improves bone density, fighting off osteoporosis and promoting overall physical function.

Beyond its physical advantages, boxing has a profound impact on mental well-being. It promotes confidence and strength, empowering you to face the challenges of menopause with resilience. Furthermore, boxing provides a healthy outlet for releasing anger and frustration, allowing you to channel your energy in a positive, empowering way. So put on your gloves, step into the ring, and discover the transformative effects of boxing on your body and mind.

Incorporating these exercises into a regular fitness routine can provide numerous benefits for women during menopause, including improved physical health, enhanced mood, better sleep, and overall well-being. However, choosing enjoyable and suitable activities for individual fitness levels is essential to maintain consistency and maximize the positive effects.

Dancing

Exercise shouldn't feel like a chore, and dancing offers a fun and engaging way to increase your heart rate and burn calories. Whether you join a dance class or dance around your living room, this activity provides numerous benefits for your body and mind. Dancing helps build muscle strength, improve flexibility, and enhance coordination. In addition, it's a versatile exercise that allows you to explore different styles like jazz, ballet, ballroom, or salsa, finding the one that resonates with you and brings you joy. Incorporating dancing into your fitness routine can make exercise more enjoyable and fulfilling while reaping the physical and mental rewards.

Yoga

Yoga is a holistic practice encompassing physical postures, breath control, and meditation, offering a comprehensive approach to managing menopausal symptoms. Research studies have shown promising results regarding the benefits of yoga for women going through menopause (Vaze & Joshi, 2010; Bapat et al., 2011) For example, integrated methods like yoga therapy have effectively reduced hot flashes and night sweats.

Additionally, even short-term yoga practice has been demonstrated to decrease psychological and physiological risk factors associated with cardiovascular disease. These findings highlight the potential of yoga as a traditional therapeutic approach to managing menopausal symptoms and promoting overall well-being. By incorporating yoga into your routine, you can experience improvements in flexibility, strength, relaxation, and mental clarity.

Tai Chi

Tai chi is a gentle and flowing martial art that offers numerous benefits for menopausal women. This mind–

body exercise focuses on slow, deliberate movements, deep breathing, and mindfulness. Regular tai chi practice improves balance, enhances bone density, boosts neurological function, and strengthens the immune system. It also addresses physiological risk factors associated with cardiovascular disease and promotes better mood, sleep quality, and overall well-being.

The meditative aspects of tai chi support the management of emotional and cognitive changes during menopause. With its holistic approach, tai chi is a valuable exercise that promotes physical health, mental well-being, and vitality during the menopausal transition.

Pilates

Pilates is a low-impact exercise method that focuses on strengthening the core muscles, improving flexibility, and enhancing overall body strength. It's particularly suitable for premenopausal and menopausal women due to its gentle nature and comprehensive benefits. Pilates exercises target various muscle groups, including the abdomen, back, hips, and buttocks, promoting better posture, balance, and muscle tone. By engaging in Pilates, women can address the specific needs associated with the premenopausal and menopausal stages of life, improve their physical well-being, and enhance their overall body strength and flexibility.

Yard or House Work

Engaging in household chores and yard work may only rarely be seen as traditional exercises, but they can provide a valuable form of physical activity. Light tasks like cleaning the floors, scrubbing the bathroom, or gardening involve dynamic movements that engage various muscle groups, such as the quads, glutes, and core.

Tackling more vigorous activities can elevate your heart rate and provide an effective aerobic workout. By incorporating these tasks into your routine, you can achieve a cleaner living space and a healthier body. If you're new to this level of physical activity, start with lighter tasks for shorter durations and gradually increase the intensity as you build stamina.

Kegels

Pelvic floor exercises, commonly known as Kegel exercises, target the muscles that support the uterus and bladder. Kegel exercises involve contracting and relaxing these muscles to improve their tone and offer several potential benefits. For example, strengthening the pelvic floor muscles can enhance sexual sensations, increasing the likelihood of achieving orgasm.

Kegel exercises may also reduce discomfort during sexual intercourse and help manage certain forms of urinary incontinence. Additionally, they can prevent or manage pelvic organ prolapse, a condition where the uterus or bladder protrudes into the vagina.

To perform Kegel exercises correctly, it's crucial to identify the correct muscles to contract and relax. While halting the urine flow during urination can help identify the pelvic floor muscles initially, it's not recommended to make this a regular practice. Instead, perform Kegel exercises with an empty bladder, holding each contraction for 2–3 seconds before releasing. As you become comfortable with the technique, aim for five sets of 10 repetitions per day, incorporating them into your daily routine while engaged in activities such as driving or sitting at your desk. By incorporating Kegel exercises into your routine, you can improve the strength and functionality of your pelvic floor muscles, leading to various benefits for your sexual and urinary health.

Join a Support Group

While the support of friends and family is invaluable, seeking a connection with other women in your community going through menopause can bring unique benefits. Engaging with a supportive network of individuals navigating the same phase in life can offer a profound sense of comfort and reassurance. Knowing you're not alone in this journey can provide a strong foundation for understanding, empathy, and shared experiences. These connections can foster a safe space for open conversations, allowing you to exchange insights, advice, and coping strategies. Building relationships with women who can relate to your experiences can bring a sense of validation and a more profound sense of community, enhancing your overall well-being during this transformative time.

Stop Smoking

It's been mentioned several times, but it can't be stressed enough: stop smoking! Women going through menopause who smoke face a higher risk of experiencing depression compared with nonsmokers. This is because smoking can exacerbate the emotional challenges that often accompany this phase of life. Moreover, it worsens many other symptoms, such as hot flashes.

If you're currently a smoker, it's highly advisable to seek assistance in quitting. Recognizing the impact of smoking on your mental health and overall well-being is an essential step toward taking control of your health during menopause. To make it easier on yourself, it's recommended to consult your doctor for guidance. They can provide valuable information about smoking-cessation resources and strategies tailored to your needs. In addition, your doctor may discuss various options with you, including nicotine replacement therapies, medications, counseling, or support groups. With their expertise and support, you can develop a personalized plan to overcome the challenges of quitting smoking and improve both your physical and mental health during the menopausal transition.

Prioritize Sleep

Sleep disturbances are a common challenge many women face during the menopausal journey. The hormonal fluctuations and physical changes during this time can disrupt your sleep patterns and leave you tired and restless. Recognizing the importance of sleep for your overall well-being, it's crucial to prioritize adequate sleep and seek strategies to improve your sleep quality.

Your doctor may advise establishing a consistent sleep schedule as part of your menopause management plan. Going to bed and waking up at the same times each day helps regulate your body's internal clock, promoting a night of more restful sleep. In addition, by sticking to a routine, your body will naturally adapt to a regular sleep pattern, making it easier to fall asleep and wake up refreshed.

Creating a sleep-friendly environment in your bedroom can also contribute to better sleep. Ensure your bedroom is dark, quiet, and cool to create a restful atmosphere. Consider using blackout curtains or an eye mask to block out unwanted light, earplugs, or a white noise machine to mask disruptive sounds and keep the temperature cool to optimize your sleep environment.

Additionally, practicing good sleep hygiene habits can further improve your sleep quality. This includes avoiding caffeine and stimulating activities close to bedtime, establishing a relaxing pre-sleep routine, and limiting exposure to electronic devices that emit blue light, which can interfere with your natural sleep–wake cycle.

If you continue to experience persistent sleep disturbances despite implementing these strategies, it's essential to consult your doctor. They can further evaluate your sleep issues, recommend additional interventions or treatments to address any underlying causes, and help get your sleep back to a more restorative and rejuvenating state. Remember, prioritizing adequate sleep is essential for maintaining your overall well-being and navigating the menopausal transition with greater resilience and vitality.

To Summarize

In conclusion, this chapter has provided valuable insights into natural remedies and lifestyle changes for managing menopause. These strategies can alleviate symptoms and enhance well-being, from nutritious diets to exercise. Remember to consult with health-care professionals and listen to your body's needs. Finally, embrace this transformative phase with confidence and grace, and empower yourself on this journey of self-discovery.

Conclusion

Throughout this transformative journey, you have embarked on a remarkable exploration of the intricate world of menopause, delving deep into its complexities and emerging with a wealth of knowledge to empower yourself during this significant phase of life. The underlying message resonating throughout this book has been crystal clear: Menopause is not simply a time of change, but an extraordinary opportunity for personal growth, self-discovery, and the cultivation of resilience.

In each chapter, we have journeyed together, unraveling different aspects of menopause to provide a comprehensive understanding. Chapter 1 served as a guiding light, illuminating the essence of menopause, unraveling its stages and symptoms, and emphasizing the utmost importance of self-care. Building upon that foundation, Chapter 2 took us on a captivating exploration of the biological processes driving menopause, revealing the intricate interplay of declining reproductive hormones and the cessation of ovulation.

With Chapter 3, we dove headfirst into HRT, thoroughly exploring this treatment option. Together, we navigated the terrain of benefits, risks, controversies, and guidelines, equipping you with the insights necessary to make informed decisions that align with your well-being. Chapter 4 then led us on an exciting journey into the realm of supplements, where we carefully examined their effectiveness, existing research, and crucial safety considerations, enabling you to make empowered choices when managing menopausal symptoms.

Transitioning to Chapter 5, we traversed the captivating landscape of herbal and natural remedies, discovering many potential benefits and carefully considering their suitability for use during this transformative phase. Then, in Chapter 6, we shifted our focus to mental health during menopause, acknowledging the profound impact of hormonal changes on our emotional well-being. We explored the causes of mood swings, anxiety, and depression, considering factors like hormonal shifts and significant life transitions.

And finally, in Chapter 7, we arrived at a destination filled with practical wisdom, emphasizing the profound significance of adopting a nutritious diet, embracing regular exercise, mastering stress management techniques, and prioritizing self-care as essential components for enhancing your overall well-being throughout menopause.

As we now approach the culmination of this enlightening journey, I urge you to take action and apply the knowledge and strategies you have gained. Embrace self-care as a daily ritual, seek guidance and support from health-care professionals who can provide personalized care, and make informed decisions that honor your unique needs and aspirations.

Furthermore, I kindly invite you to share your valuable feedback by leaving a review wherever you purchased this book. Your insights and experiences will contribute to the ongoing improvement of this work and serve as a guiding light for other individuals seeking knowledge and empowerment on their menopause journey. By spreading the word and sharing this invaluable resource, you can make a meaningful impact in the lives of those navigating menopause, empowering them to embrace this transformative phase with confidence and vitality.

Thank you wholeheartedly for embarking on this extraordinary exploration of menopause. May you now stride forward with renewed confidence, embracing the limitless possibilities that await you and crafting a life of vibrancy and fulfillment during this transformative phase and beyond.

References

Are You Getting Enough Sleep? (2022, September 19). Centers for Disease Control and Prevention. https://www.cdc.gov/sleep/features/getting-enough-sleep.html

Asian Ginseng. (2020, August). National Center for Complementary and Alternative Medicine. https://www.nccih.nih.gov/health/asian-ginseng

Atkinson, C., Compston, J. E., Day, N. E., Dowsett, M., & Bingham, S. A. (2004). The effects of phytoestrogen isoflavones on bone density in women: A double-blind, randomized, placebo-controlled trial. *The American Journal of Clinical Nutrition,* *79*(2), 326–333. https://doi.org/10.1093/ajcn/79.2.326

Avis, N. E., Crawford, S. L., Greendale, G., Bromberger, J. T., Everson-Rose, S. A., Gold, E. B., Hess, R., Joffe, H., Kravitz, H. M., Tepper, P. G., & Thurston, R. C.; for the Study of Women's Health Across the Nation (SWAN). (2015). Duration of menopausal vasomotor symptoms over the menopause transition. *JAMA Internal Medicine,* *175*(4), 531. https://doi.org/10.1001/jamainternmed.2014.8063

Babio, N., Toledo, E., Estruch, R., Ros, E., Martínez-González, M. A., Castañer, O., Bulló, M., Corella, D., Arós, F., Gómez-Gracia, E., Ruiz-Gutiérrez, V., Fiol, M., Lapetra, J., Lamuela-Raventos, R. M., Serra-Majem, L., Pintó, X., Basora, J., Sorlí, J. V., & Salas-Salvadó, J.; for the PREDIMED Study Investigators. (2014). Mediterranean diets and metabolic syndrome status in the PREDIMED randomized trial. *Canadian Medical Association Journal = Journal de l'Association Medicale Canadienne, 186*(17), E649–57. https://doi.org/10.1503/cmaj.140764

Bani, S., Hasanpour, S., Farzad Rik, L., Hasankhani, H., & Sharami, S. H. (2013). The effect of folic acid on menopausal hot flashes: A randomized clinical trial. *Journal of Caring Sciences, 2*(2), 131–140. https://doi.org/10.5681/jcs.2013.016

Bapat, D., Deshmukh, U., Joshi, S., & Khandwe, R. (2011). Effect of yoga on menopausal symptoms. *Menopause International, 17*(3), 78–81. https://doi.org/10.1258/mi.2011.011020

Barnard, N. D., Scialli, A. R., Turner-McGrievy, G., Lanou, A. J., & Glass, J. (2005). The effects of a low-fat, plant-based dietary intervention on body weight, metabolism, and insulin sensitivity. *The American Journal of Medicine, 118*(9), 991–997. https://doi.org/10.1016/j.amjmed.2005.03.039

Barton, D. L., Schroeder, K. C. F., Banerjee, T., Wolf, S., Keith, T., & Elkins, G. (2017). Efficacy of a biobehavioral intervention for hot flashes: A randomized controlled pilot study. *Menopause,*

24(7), 774–782. https://doi.org/10.1097/GME.0000000000000837

Beezhold, B., Radnitz, C., McGrath, R. E., & Feldman, A. (2018). Vegans report less bothersome vasomotor and physical menopausal symptoms than omnivores. *Maturitas*, *112*, 12–17. https://doi.org/10.1016/j.maturitas.2018.03.009

Beharry, S., & Heinrich, M. (2018). Is the hype around the reproductive health claims of maca (*Lepidium meyenii* Walp.) justified? *Journal of Ethnopharmacology*, *211*, 126–170. https://doi.org/10.1016/j.jep.2017.08.003

Black Cohosh. (2020). National Institutes of Health—Office of Dietary Supplements. https://ods.od.nih.gov/factsheets/BlackCohosh-HealthProfessional/

Boschmann, M., Steiniger, J., Hille, U., Tank, J., Adams, F., Sharma, A. M., Klaus, S., Luft, F. C., & Jordan, J. (2003). Water-induced thermogenesis. *The Journal of Clinical Endocrinology & Metabolism*, *88*(12), 6015–6019. https://doi.org/10.1210/jc.2003-030780

Brazier, Y. (2017, March 20). *Aromatherapy: What you need to know.* Medical News Today. https://www.medicalnewstoday.com/articles/10884

Bromberger, J. T., & Kravitz, H. M. (2011). Mood and menopause: Findings from the study of women's health across the nation (SWAN) over ten years. *Obstetrics and Gynecology Clinics of North America*, *38*(3), 609–625. https://doi.org/10.1016/j.ogc.2011.05.011

Brooks, N. A., Wilcox, G., Walker, K. Z., Ashton, J. F., Cox, M. B., & Stojanovska, L. Beneficial effects of *Lepidium meyenii* (maca) on psychological symptoms and measures of sexual dysfunction in postmenopausal women are not related to estrogen or androgen content. *Menopause*, *15*(6), 1157–1162. https://doi.org/10.1097/gme.0b013e3181732953

Brown, M. J. (2023, April). *11 natural remedies for menopause relief.* Healthline. https://www.healthline.com/nutrition/11-natural-menopause-tips

Cagnacci, A., & Venier, M. (2019). The controversial history of hormone replacement therapy. *Medicina*, *55*(9), 602. https://doi.org/10.3390/medicina55090602

Calcium. (2022, October 6). National Institutes of Health—Office of Dietary Supplements. https://ods.od.nih.gov/factsheets/Calcium-HealthProfessional/

Cappelloni, L. (2017, November 22). *The Best Activities to Do During Menopause.* Healthline.

https://www.healthline.com/health/ten-best-menopause-activities

Caretto, M., Giannini, A., & Simoncini, T. (2019). An integrated approach to diagnosing and managing sleep disorders in menopausal women. *Maturitas*, *128*, 1–3. https://doi.org/10.1016/j.maturitas.2019.06.008

Cetisli, N. E., Saruhan, A., & Kivcak, B. & (2015). The effects of flaxseed on menopausal symptoms and quality of life. *Holistic Nursing Practice*, *29*(3), 151–157. https://doi.org/10.1097/hnp.00000000000000085

Chasteberry. (2020, July). National Center for Complementary and Integrative Health. https://www.nccih.nih.gov/health/chasteberry

Chen, L.-R., Ko, N.-Y., & Chen, K.-H. (2019). Isoflavone supplements for menopausal women: A systematic review. *Nutrients*, *11*(11), 2649. https://doi.org/10.3390/nu11112649

Chen, M., Lin, C., & Liu, C. (2014). Efficacy of phytoestrogens for menopausal symptoms: A meta-analysis and systematic review. *Climacteric*, *18*(2), 260–269. https://doi.org/10.3109/13697137.2014.966241

Cherney, K. (2020, June 5). *Effects of menopause on the body*. Healthline.

https://www.healthline.com/health/menopaus
e/hrt-effects-on-body

Chlebowski, R. T., Rohan, T. E., Manson, J. E., Aragaki,
A. K., Kaunitz, A., Stefanick, M. L., Simon, M.
S., Johnson, K. C., Wactawski-Wende, J.,
O'Sullivan, M. J., Adams-Campbell, L. L., Nassir,
R., Lessin, L. S., & Prentice, R. L. (2015). Breast
cancer after use of estrogen plus progestin and
estrogen alone. *JAMA Oncology, 1*(3), 296.
https://doi.org/10.1001/jamaoncol.2015.0494

Chopra, S., Sharma, K. A., Ranjan, P., Malhotra, A.,
Kumari, A., & Vikram, N. K. (2019). Weight
management module for perimenopausal
women: A practical guide for gynecologists.
Journal of Mid-Life Health, *10*(4), 165.
https://doi.org/10.4103/jmh.jmh_155_19

Clayton, A. H., & Ninan, P. T. (2010). Depression or
menopause? Presentation and management of
major depressive disorder in perimenopausal and
postmenopausal women. *The Primary Care
Companion for CNS Disorders*.
https://doi.org/10.4088/pcc.08r00747blu

Clifton-Bligh, P. B., Baber, R. J., Fulcher, G. R., Nery,
M.-L., & Moreton, T. (2001). The effect of
isoflavones extracted from red clover (rimostil)
on lipid and bone metabolism. *Menopause, 8*(4),
259–265. https://doi.org/10.1097/00042192-
200107000-00007

Cramer, H., Lauche, R., Langhorst, J., & Dobos, G.
(2012). Effectiveness of yoga for menopausal

symptoms: A systematic review and meta-analysis of randomized controlled trials. *Evidence-Based Complementary and Alternative Medicine, 2012,* 863905. https://doi.org/10.1155/2012/863905

Cramer, H., Peng, W., & Lauche, R. (2018). Yoga for menopausal symptoms—A systematic review and meta-analysis. *Maturitas, 109,* 13–25. https://doi.org/10.1016/j.maturitas.2017.12.005

Dąbrowska-Galas, M., Dąbrowska, J., Ptaszkowski, K., & Plinta, R. (2019). High physical activity level may reduce menopausal symptoms. *Medicina, 55*(8), 466. https://doi.org/10.3390/medicina55080466

Darsareh, F., Taavoni, S., Joolaee, S., & Haghani, H. (2012). Effect of aromatherapy massage on menopausal symptoms. *Menopause: The Journal of the North American Menopause Society, 19*(9), 995–999. https://doi.org/10.1097/gme.0b013e318248ea16

Davy, B. M., Dennis, E. A., Dengo, A. L., Wilson, K. L., & Davy, K. P. (2008). Water consumption reduces energy intake at a breakfast meal in obese older adults. *Journal of the American Dietetic Association, 108*(7), 1236–1239. https://doi.org/10.1016/j.jada.2008.04.013

Debice, S. P. (2021, January 31). *Is your post-menopausal fatigue due to iron deficient anaemia?* Inspired Health. https://inspiredhealth.co.uk/blogs/the-menopause-blog/is-your-post-menopausal-fatigue-due-to-iron-deficient-anaemia

Depression & Menopause. (n.d.). North American Menopause Society. https://www.menopause.org/for-women/menopauseflashes/mental-health-at-menopause/depression-menopause

Dew, T. P., & Williamson, G. (2013). Controlled flax interventions for the improvement of menopausal symptoms and postmenopausal bone health. *Menopause, 20*(11), 1207–1215. https://doi.org/10.1097/gme.0b013e3182896ae5

Dong Quai. (2006). PubMed; National Institute of Child Health and Human Development. https://pubmed.ncbi.nlm.nih.gov/30000896/

Dresden, D. (2021, December 23). *Menopause supplements: Effectiveness, side effects, and safety.* Medical News Today. https://www.medicalnewstoday.com/articles/menopause-supplements#black-cohosh

Emamverdikhan , A. P., Golmakani, N., Tabassi , S. AS., Hassanzadeh, M., Sharifi, N., & Shakeri, M. T. (2016). A survey of the therapeutic effects of vitamin E suppositories on vaginal atrophy in postmenopausal women. *Iranian Journal of Nursing and Midwifery Research, 21*(5), 475. https://doi.org/10.4103/1735-9066.193393

The Emotional Roller Coaster of Menopause. (2023, April 7). WebMD. https://www.webmd.com/menopause/guide/emotional-roller-coaster

Ertel, K. A., Glymour, M. M., & Berkman, L. F. (2008). Effects of social integration on preserving memory function in a nationally representative US elderly population. *American Journal of Public Health*, *98*(7), 1215–1220. https://doi.org/10.2105/AJPH.2007.113654

Estrogen Vaginal. (n.d.). Medline Plus. https://medlineplus.gov/druginfo/meds/a606005.html

Evening Primrose Oil. (n.d.). National Center for Complementary and Integrative Health. https://www.nccih.nih.gov/health/evening-primrose-oil

The Experts Do Agree About Hormone Therapy. (n.d.). North American Menopause Society, American Society for Reproductive Medicine, & Endocrine Society. https://www.menopause.org/docs/for-women/expertsagree_consumer.pdf?sfvrsn=4

Farzaneh, F., Fatehi, S., Sohrabi, M.-R., & Alizadeh, K. (2013). The effect of oral evening primrose oil on menopausal hot flashes: A randomized clinical trial. *Archives of Gynecology and Obstetrics*, *288*(5), 1075–1079. https://doi.org/10.1007/s00404-013-2852-6

Franco, O. H., Chowdhury, R., Troup, J., Voortman, T., Kunutsor, S., Kavousi, M., Oliver-Williams, C., & Muka, T. (2016). Use of plant-based therapies and menopausal symptoms. *JAMA*, *315*(23), 2554–2563. https://doi.org/10.1001/jama.2016.8012

Gangwisch, J. E., Hale, L., Garcia, L., Malaspina, D., Opler, M. G., Payne, M. E., Rossom, R. C., & Lane, D. (2015). High glycemic index diet as a risk factor for depression: Analyses from the Women's Health Initiative. *The American Journal of Clinical Nutrition*, *102*(2), 454–463. https://doi.org/10.3945/ajcn.114.103846

Gardener, H., Wright, C. B., Dong, C., Cheung, K., DeRosa, J., Nannery, M., Stern, Y., Elkind, M. S. V., & Sacco, R. L. (2016). Ideal cardiovascular health and cognitive aging in the Northern Manhattan Study. *Journal of the American Heart Association*, *5*(3), e002731. https://doi.org/10.1161/jaha.115.002731

Geller, S. E., & Studee, L. (2005). Botanical and dietary supplements for menopausal symptoms: What works, what does not. *Journal of Women's Health*, *14*(7), 634–649. https://doi.org/10.1089/jwh.2005.14.634

Genazzani, A. R., Monteleone, P., Giannini, A., & Simoncini, T. (2021). Hormone therapy in the postmenopausal years: Considering benefits and risks in clinical practice. *Human Reproduction Update*, *27*(6), 1115–1150. https://doi.org/10.1093/humupd/dmab026

Ghazanfarpour, M., Sadeghi, R., Roudsari, R. L., Khorsand , Khadivzadeh, T., & I., Muoio, B. (2016). Red clover for treatment of hot flashes and menopausal symptoms: A systematic review and meta-analysis. *Journal of Obstetrics and Gynaecology*, *36*(3), 301–311. https://doi.org/10.3109/01443615.2015.10492 49

Gordon, J. L., Nowakowski, S., & Gurvich, C. (2022). Editorial: The psychology of menopause. *Frontiers in Global Women's Health*, *2*. https://doi.org/10.3389/fgwh.2021.828676

Goss, A. M., Chandler-Laney, P. C., Ovalle, F., Goree, L. L., Azziz, R., Desmond, R. A., Wright Bates, G., & Gower, B. A. (2014). Effects of a eucaloric reduced-carbohydrate diet on body composition and fat distribution in women with PCOS. *Metabolism*, *63*(10), 1257–1264. https://doi.org/10.1016/j.metabol.2014.07.007

Gougeon, L., Payette, H., Morais, J. A., Gaudreau, P., Shatenstein, B., & Gray-Donald, K. (2015). Intakes of folate, vitamin B6 and B12 and risk of depression in community-dwelling older adults: The Quebec Longitudinal Study On Nutrition And Aging. *European Journal of Clinical Nutrition*, *70*(3), 380–385. https://doi.org/10.1038/ejcn.2015.202

Gower, B. A., & Goss, A. M. (2014). A lower-carbohydrate, higher-fat diet reduces abdominal and intermuscular fat and increases insulin sensitivity in adults at risk of type 2 diabetes. *The*

Journal of Nutrition, *145*(1), 177S183S. https://doi.org/10.3945/jn.114.195065

Grantham, J. P., & Henneberg, M. (2014). The estrogen hypothesis of obesity. *PLoS ONE*, *9*(6). https://doi.org/10.1371/journal.pone.0099776

Grey, A., Garg, S., Dray, M., Purvis, L., Horne, A., Callon, K., Gamble, G., Bolland, M., Reid, I. R., & Cundy, T. (2013). Low-dose fluoride in postmenopausal women: A randomized controlled trial. *The Journal of Clinical Endocrinology & Metabolism*, *98*(6), 2301–2307. https://doi.org/10.1210/jc.2012-4062

Hardcastle, A. C., Aucott, L., Fraser, W. D., Reid, D. M., & Macdonald, H. M. (2010). Dietary patterns, bone resorption and bone mineral density in early post-menopausal Scottish women. *European Journal of Clinical Nutrition*, *65*(3), 378–385. https://doi.org/10.1038/ejcn.2010.264

Henderson, V. W., & Lobo, R. A. (2012). Hormone therapy and the risk of stroke: Perspectives 10 years after the Women's Health Initiative Trials. *Climacteric*, *15*(3), 229–234. https://doi.org/10.3109/13697137.2012.65625 4

Hill, A. (2020, September 30). *10 Herbs and Supplements for Menopause.* Healthline. https://www.healthline.com/nutrition/menopa use-herbs

Holland, K. (2020, August 12). *Mental Health, Depression, and Menopause.* Healthline. https://www.healthline.com/health/menopaus e/mental-health

Hormone Replacement Therapy (HRT). (2019, September 9). National Health Service. https://www.nhs.uk/conditions/hormone-replacement-therapy-hrt/

Hormone Replacement Therapy (HRT). (2022, November 3). NHS Inform. https://www.nhsinform.scot/tests-and-treatments/medicines-and-medical-aids/types-of-medicine/hormone-replacement-therapy-hrt

Hormone Replacement Therapy for Menopause. (2021, October 13). WebMD. https://www.webmd.com/menopause/guide/ menopause-hormone-therapy

Hormone Therapy for Menopause Symptoms. (2021, June 28). Cleveland Clinic. https://my.clevelandclinic.org/health/treatmen ts/15245-hormone-therapy-for-menopause-symptoms

Hot Flashes: What Can I Do? (2021, September 30). National Institute on Aging. https://www.nia.nih.gov/health/hot-flashes-what-can-i-do

How Much Physical Activity Do Adults Need? (2022, June 2). Centers for Disease Control and Prevention.

https://www.cdc.gov/physicalactivity/basics/a
dults/index.htm

Huang, A. J., Subak, L. L., Wing, R., West, D. S.,
Hernandez, A. L., Macer, J., & Grady, D.;
Program to Reduce Incontinence by Diet and
Exercise Investigators (2010). An intensive
behavioral weight loss intervention and hot
flushes in women. *Archives of Internal Medicine*,
170(13), 1161.
https://doi.org/10.1001/archinternmed.2010.1
62

Iftikhar, N. (2018, June 19). *Treating Menopause With
Antidepressants.* Healthline.
https://www.healthline.com/health/antidepres
sants-for-menopause

Imam, B., Aziz, K., Khan, M., Zubair, T., & Iqbal, A.
(2019). Role of bisphosphonates in
postmenopausal women with osteoporosis to
prevent future fractures: A literature review.
Cureus, *11*(8), e5328.
https://doi.org/10.7759/cureus.5328

Innes, K. E., Selfe, T. K., & Vishnu, A. (2010). Mind-
body therapies for menopausal symptoms: A
systematic review. *Maturitas*, *66*(2), 135–149.
https://doi.org/10.1016/j.maturitas.2010.01.01
6

Jenabi, E., Shobeiri, F., Hazavehei, S. M. M., &
Roshanaei, G. (2017). The effect of valerian on
the severity and frequency of hot flashes: A
triple-blind randomized clinical trial. *Women &*

Health, *58*(3), 297–304. https://doi.org/10.1080/03630242.2017.12960 58

Joffe, H., Guthrie, K. A., LaCroix, A. Z., Reed, S. D., Ensrud, K. E., Manson, J. E., Newton, K. M., Freeman, E. W., Anderson, G. L., Larson, J. C., Hunt, J., Shifren, J., Rexrode, K. M., Caan, B., Sternfeld, B., Carpenter, J. S., & Cohen, L. (2014). Low-dose estradiol and the serotonin-norepinephrine reuptake inhibitor venlafaxine for vasomotor symptoms. *JAMA Internal Medicine*, *174*(7), 1058. https://doi.org/10.1001/jamainternmed.2014.1 891

Johnson, A., Roberts, L., & Elkins, G. (2019). Complementary and alternative medicine for menopause. *Journal of Evidence-Based Integrative Medicine*, *24*, 2515690X1982938. https://doi.org/10.1177/2515690x19829380

Johnston, B. C., Kanters, S., Bandayrel, K., Wu, P., Naji, P. F., Siemieniuk, R. A., Ball, G. D. C., Busse, J. W., Thorlund, K., Guyatt, G., Jansen, J., & Mills, E. J. (2014). Comparison of weight loss among named diet programs in overweight and obese adults. *JAMA*, *312*(9), 923. https://doi.org/10.1001/jama.2014.10397

Kandola, A. (2023, May 15). *What Are the Health Benefits of Wild Yam?* Medical News Today. https://www.medicalnewstoday.com/articles/3 22423#benefits-and-uses

Komesaroff, P. A., Black, C. V., Cable, V., & Sudhir, K. (2001). Effects of wild yam extract on menopausal symptoms, lipids and sex hormones in healthy menopausal women. *Climacteric, 4*(2), 144–150. https://pubmed.ncbi.nlm.nih.gov/11428178/

Kong, A., Beresford, S. A. A., Alfano, C. M., Foster-Schubert, K. E., Neuhouser, M. L., Johnson, D. B., Duggan, C., Wang, C.-Y., Xiao, L., Jeffery, R. W., Bain, C. E., & McTiernan, A. (2012). Self-monitoring and eating-related behaviors are associated with 12-month weight loss in postmenopausal overweight-to-obese women. *Journal of the Academy of Nutrition and Dietetics, 112*(9), 1428–1435. https://doi.org/10.1016/j.jand.2012.05.014

Křížová, L., Dadáková, K., Kašparovská, J., & Kašparovský, T. (2019). Isoflavones. *Molecules, 24*(6), 1076. https://doi.org/10.3390/molecules24061076

Kroenke, C. H., Caan, B. J, Stefanick, M. L., Anderson, G., Brzyski, R., Johnson, K. C., LeBlanc, E., Lee, C., La Croix, A, Z., Park, H. L., Sims, S. T., Vitolins, M., & Wallace, R. (2012). Effects of a dietary intervention and weight change on vasomotor symptoms in the Women's Health Initiative. *Menopause (New York, N.Y.), 19*(9), 980–988. https://doi.org/10.1097/gme.0b013e31824f606e

Leach, M. J., & Moore, V. (2012). Black cohosh (*Cimicifuga* spp.) for menopausal symptoms. *Cochrane Database of Systematic Reviews*, *9*. https://doi.org/10.1002/14651858.cd007244.pub2

LeBlanc, E. S., Hedlin, H., Qin, F., Desai, M., Wactawski-Wende, J., Perrin, N., Manson, J. E., Johnson, K. C., Masaki, K., Tylavsky, F. A., & Stefanick, M. L. (2015). Calcium and vitamin D supplementation do not influence menopause-related symptoms: Results of the women's health initiative trial. *Maturitas*, *81*(3), 377–383. https://doi.org/10.1016/j.maturitas.2015.04.007

Lee, H. W., Choi, J., Lee, Y., Kil, K.-J., & Lee, M. S. (2016). Ginseng for managing menopausal woman's health. *Medicine*, *95*(38), e4914. https://doi.org/10.1097/md.0000000000004914

Lee, M. S., Shin, B.-C., Yang, E. J., Lim, H.-J., & Ernst, E. (2011). Maca (*Lepidium meyenii*) for treatment of menopausal symptoms: A systematic review. *Maturitas*, *70*(3), 227–233. https://doi.org/10.1016/j.maturitas.2011.07.017

Levis, S., & Griebeler, M. L. (2010). The role of soy foods in the treatment of menopausal symptoms123. *The Journal of Nutrition*, *140*(12), 2318S2321S. https://doi.org/10.3945/jn.110.124388

Lisabeth, L., & Bushnell, C. (2012). Stroke risk in women: the role of menopause and hormone therapy. *The Lancet Neurology, 11*(1), 82–91. https://doi.org/10.1016/s1474-4422(11)70269-1

MacLennan, A. H., Henderson , V. W., Paine, B. J., Mathias, J., Ramsay, E. N., Ryan, P., Stocks, N. P., & Taylor, A. W. (2006). Hormone therapy, timing of initiation, and cognition in women aged older than 60 years: The REMEMBER pilot study. *Menopause, 13*(1), 28–36. https://doi.org/10.1097/01.gme.0000191204.38664.61

Mahon, A. K., Flynn, M. G., Stewart, L. K., McFarlin, B. K., Iglay, H. B., Mattes, R. D., Lyle, R. M., Considine, R. V., & Campbell, W. W. (2007). Protein intake during energy restriction: Effects on body composition and markers of metabolic and cardiovascular health in postmenopausal women. *Journal of the American College of Nutrition, 26*(2), 182–189. https://doi.org/10.1080/07315724.2007.10719600

Mancini, J. G., Filion, K. B., Atallah, R., & Eisenberg, M. J. (2016). Systematic review of the Mediterranean diet for long-term weight loss. *The American Journal of Medicine, 129*(4), 407–415.e4. https://doi.org/10.1016/j.amjmed.2015.11.028

Mayo Clinic Staff. *Fitness Tips for Menopause: Why Fitness Counts.* (2022, December 3). Mayo Clinic. https://www.mayoclinic.org/healthy-lifestyle/womens-health/in-depth/fitness-tips-for-menopause/art-20044602

Mayo Clinic Staff. *Hormone Therapy: Is It Right For You?* (2022, December 6). Mayo Clinic. https://www.mayoclinic.org/diseases-conditions/menopause/in-depth/hormone-therapy/ART-20046372

Mellberg, C., Sandberg, S., Ryberg, M., Eriksson, M., Brage, S., Larsson , C., Olsson, T., & Lindahl, B. (2014). Long-term effects of a Palaeolithic-type diet in obese postmenopausal women: a 2-year randomized trial. *European Journal of Clinical Nutrition*, *68*(3), 350–357. https://doi.org/10.1038/ejcn.2013.290

Menopausal Symptoms: In Depth. (2017, May). National Center for Complementary and Integrative Health. https://www.nccih.nih.gov/health/menopausal-symptoms-in-depth

Menopause. (2023, May 25). Mayo Clinic. https://www.mayoclinic.org/diseases-conditions/menopause/symptoms-causes/syc-20353397

Menopause and Mental Health. (2020, March 1). Harvard Health. https://www.health.harvard.edu/womens-health/menopause-and-mental-health

Menopause and Your Mental Wellbeing. (2022, November 29). NHS Inform.

https://www.nhsinform.scot/healthy-living/womens-health/later-years-around-50-years-and-over/menopause-and-post-menopause-health/menopause-and-your-mental-wellbeing

Menopause Symptoms and Relief. (2021, February 22). Office on Women's Health, U.S. Department of Health & Human Services. https://www.womenshealth.gov/menopause/menopause-symptoms-and-relief

Menopause Treatment. (2021, February 22). Office on Women's Health, U.S. Department of Health & Human Services. https://www.womenshealth.gov/menopause/menopause-treatment

Milart, P., Woźniakowska, E., & Wrona, W. (2018). Selected vitamins and quality of life in menopausal women. *Menopause Review, 17*(4), 180–184. https://doi.org/10.5114/pm.2018.81742

Minelli, C., Abrams, K. R., Sutton, A. J., & Cooper, N. J. (2004). Benefits and harms associated with hormone replacement therapy: clinical decision analysis. *BMJ, 328*(7436), 371. https://doi.org/10.1136/bmj.328.7436.371

Mirabi, P., & Mojab, F. (2013). The effects of valerian root on hot flashes in menopausal women. *Iranian Journal of Pharmaceutical Research: IJPR, 12*(1), 217–222. https://pubmed.ncbi.nlm.nih.gov/24250592/

Mumusoglu, S., & Yildiz, B. O. (2019). Metabolic syndrome during menopause. *Current Vascular Pharmacology*, *17*(6), 595–603. https://doi.org/10.2174/1570161116666180904094149

Muhleisen, A. L., & Herbst-Kralovetz, M. M. (2016). Menopause and the vaginal microbiome. *Maturitas*, *91*, 42–50. https://doi.org/10.1016/j.maturitas.2016.05.015

Naseri, R., Farnia, V., Yazdchi, K., Alikhani, M., Basanj, B., & Salemi, S. (2019). Comparison of *vitex agnus-castus* extracts with placebo in reducing menopausal symptoms: A randomized double-blind study. *Korean Journal of Family Medicine*, *40*(6), 362–367. https://doi.org/10.4082/kjfm.18.0067

Nguyen, M.-L. (2013). The use of pregabalin in the treatment of hot flashes. *Canadian Pharmacists Journal / Revue Des Pharmaciens Du Canada*, *146*(4), 193–196. https://doi.org/10.1177/1715163513490636*Menopause*. (2021, October 5). Cleveland Clinic. https://my.clevelandclinic.org/health/diseases/21841-menopause

O'Donnell, S., Cranney, A., Wells, G. A., Adachi, J., & Reginster, J-Y. (2006, October 18). *Strontium ranelate for osteoporosis in women after menopause.* Cochrane.org. https://www.cochrane.org/CD005326/MUSK

EL_strontium-ranelate-osteoporosis-women-after-menopause

Osteoporosis. (2021, February 9). Office on Women's Health, U.S. Department of Health & Human Services. https://www.womenshealth.gov/a-z-topics/osteoporosis

Petrikovsky, B. M. (2019). Individual approach to hormone replacement therapy – A computer assisted method of assessment of the minimal useful dose. *American Journal of Biomedical Science & Research*, *1*(1), 26–28. https://biomedgrid.com/fulltext/volume1/individual-approach-to-hormone-replacement-therapy-a-computer-assisted-method-of-assessment-of-the-minimal-useful-dose.ID.000507.php

Phaniendra, A., Jestadi, D. B., & Periyasamy, L. (2014). Free radicals: Properties, sources, targets, and their implication in various diseases. *Indian Journal of Clinical Biochemistry*, *30*(1), 11–26. https://doi.org/10.1007/s12291-014-0446-0

Pinkerton, J. V., Joffe, H., Kazempour, K., Mekonnen, H., Bhaskar, S., & Lippman, J. (2015). Low-dose paroxetine (7.5 mg) improves sleep in women with vasomotor symptoms associated with menopause. *Menopause*, *22*(1), 50–58. https://doi.org/10.1097/gme.0000000000000311

Prior, J. C. (2011). Progesterone for symptomatic perimenopause treatment - progesterone politics, physiology and potential for perimenopause. *Facts, Views & Vision in ObGyn*, *3*(2), 109–120. https://pubmed.ncbi.nlm.nih.gov/24753856/

Railton, D. (2023, May 12). *Do Vitamins Help With Menopause?* Medical News Today. https://www.medicalnewstoday.com/articles/3 17864

Ratner, S., & Ofri, D. (2001). Menopause and hormone-replacement therapy. *Western Journal of Medicine*, *175*(1), 32–34. https://www.ncbi.nlm.nih.gov/pmc/articles/P MC1071462/

Red Clover. (2020, October). National Center for Complementary and Integrative Health, U.S. Department of Health & Human Services. https://www.nccih.nih.gov/health/red-clover

Richards, L. (2021, January 29). 9 *Foods High in Phytoestrogens.* Medical News Today. https://www.medicalnewstoday.com/articles/f oods-high-in-estrogen#beneficial

Rietjens, I. M. C. M., Louisse, J., & Beekmann, K. (2016). The potential health effects of dietary phytoestrogens. *British Journal of Pharmacology*, *174*(11), 1263–1280. https://doi.org/10.1111/bph.13622

Roberts, H., & Hickey , M. (2016). Managing the menopause: An update. *Maturitas, 86*, 53–58.

https://doi.org/10.1016/j.maturitas.2016.01.00
7

Rössler, W., Ajdacic-Gross, V., Riecher-Rössler, A., Angst, J., & Hengartner, M. P. (2016). Does menopausal transition really influence mental health? Findings from the prospective long-term Zurich study. *World Psychiatry, 15*(2), 146–154. https://doi.org/10.1002/wps.20319

Sayón-Orea, C., Santiago, S., Cuervo , M., Martínez-González, M. A., Garcia , A., & Martínez, J. A. (2015). Adherence to Mediterranean dietary pattern and menopausal symptoms in relation to overweight/obesity in Spanish perimenopausal and postmenopausal women. *Menopause, 22*(7), 750–757. https://doi.org/10.1097/gme.00000000000003 78

Selective Estrogen Receptor Modulators (SERMS). (2023, February 3). Cleveland Clinic. https://my.clevelandclinic.org/health/treatmen ts/24732-selective-estrogen-receptor-modulators-serm

Shifren, J. L., & Gass, M. L. S.; for the NAMS Recommendations for Clinical Care of Midlife Women Working Group. (2014). The North American Menopause Society recommendations for clinical care of midlife women. *Menopause, 21*(10), 1038–1062. https://doi.org/10.1097/gme.00000000000003 19

Shin, B.-C., Lee, M. S., Yang, E. J., Lim, H.-S., & Ernst, E. (2010). Maca (*L. meyenii*) for improving sexual function: A systematic review. *BMC Complementary and Alternative Medicine, 10*(1). https://doi.org/10.1186/1472-6882-10-44

Singh, B., Olds, T., Curtis, R., Dumuid, D., Virgara, R., Watson, A., Szeto, K., O'Connor, E., Ferguson, T., Eglitis, E., Miatke, A., Simpson, C. E., & Maher, C. (2023). Effectiveness of physical activity interventions for improving depression, anxiety and distress: An overview of systematic reviews. *British Journal of Sports Medicine, 1*(1). https://doi.org/10.1136/bjsports-2022-106195

Song, S.-W., Kim, H.-N., Shim, J.-Y., Yoo, B.-Y., Kim, D.-H., Lee, S.-H., Park, J.-S., Kim, M.-J., Yoo, J.-H. Cho, B., Kang, H.-C., Kim, K.-M., Kim, S.-S., & Kim, K.-S. (2018). Safety and tolerability of Korean red ginseng in healthy adults: A multicenter, double-blind, randomized, placebo-controlled trial. *Journal of Ginseng Research, 42*(4), 571–576. https://doi.org/10.1016/j.jgr.2018.07.002

Sood, R., Faubion, S., Kuhle, C., Thielen, J., & Shuster, L. (2014). Prescribing menopausal hormone therapy: An evidence-based approach. *International Journal of Women's Health, 6*, 47–57. https://doi.org/10.2147/ijwh.s38342*Soy*. (2020, December). National Center for Complementary and Alternative Medicine, U.S. Department of Health & Human Services. https://www.nccih.nih.gov/health/soy

Spritzler, F. (2023, March 14). *How to Lose Weight Around Menopause (And Keep It Off)*. Healthline. https://www.healthline.com/nutrition/lose-weight-in-menopause

Stelter, G. (2018, May 8). 5 *Pilates Moves for Menopause*. Healthline. https://www.healthline.com/health/pilates-moves-for-menopause

Sternfeld, B., Guthrie, K. A., Kristine E. E., LaCroix, A. Z., Larson, J, C., Dunn, A. L., Anderson, G. L., Seguin, R. A., Carpenter, J. S., Newton, K. M., Reed, S. D., Freeman, E. W., Cohen, L. S., Joffe, H., Roberts, M., & Caan, B. J. (2013). Efficacy of exercise for menopausal symptoms. *Menopause, 21*(4), 1. https://doi.org/10.1097/gme.0b013e31829e4089

Strontium Ranelate. (n.d.) ScienceDirect. https://www.sciencedirect.com/topics/medicine-and-dentistry/strontium-ranelate

Supplements for Menopause Symptoms: Are They Safe? (2022, October 26). Cleveland Clinic. https://health.clevelandclinic.org/menopause-supplements/

Taavoni, S., Nazem Ekbatani, N., & Haghani, H. (2013). Valerian/lemon balm use for sleep disorders during menopause. *Complementary Therapies in Clinical Practice, 19*(4), 193–196. https://doi.org/10.1016/j.ctcp.2013.07.002

Talaulikar, V. (2022). Menopause transition: Physiology and symptoms. *Best Practice & Research Clinical Obstetrics & Gynaecology*, *81*. https://doi.org/10.1016/j.bpobgyn.2022.03.003

Tepper, P. G, Brooks, M. M., Randolph, J. F. Jr., Crawford, S. L., El Khoudary, S, R., Gold, E, B., Lasley, B. L., Jones, B., Joffe, H., Hess, R., Avis, N. E., Harlow, S., McConnell, D. S., Bromberger, J. T., Zheng, H., Ruppert, K., & Thurston, R. C. Characterizing the trajectories of vasomotor symptoms across the menopausal transition. *Menopause*, *23*(10), 1067–1074. https://doi.org/10.1097/gme.00000000000006 76

Te Morenga, L. A., Levers, M. T., Williams, S. M., Brown, R. C., & Mann, M. J. (2011). Comparison of high protein and high fiber weight-loss diets in women with risk factors for the metabolic syndrome: A randomized trial. *Nutrition Journal*, *10*, 40. https://doi.org/10.1186/1475-2891-10-40

Thompson, H. J., Sedlacek, S. M., Playdon, M. C., Wolfe, P. McGinley, J. N., Paul, D., & Lakoski, S. G. (2015). Weight loss interventions for breast cancer survivors: Impact of dietary pattern. *PLOS ONE*, *10*(5), e0127366. https://doi.org/10.1371/journal.pone.0127366

Turner-McGrievy, G. M., Barnard, N. D., & Scialli, A. R. (2012). A two-year randomized weight loss trial comparing a vegan diet to a more moderate low-fat diet. *Obesity*, *15*(9), 2276–2281. https://doi.org/10.1038/oby.2007.270

Valerian. (2013, March 15). National Institutes of Health Office of Dietary Supplements, U.S. Department of Health & Human Services. https://ods.od.nih.gov/factsheets/Valerian-HealthProfessional/

van Die, M. D., Burger, H. G., Bone, K. M., Cohen, M. M., & Teede, H. J. (2009). *Hypericum perforatum* with *Vitex agnus-castus* in menopausal symptoms. *Menopause*, *16*(1), 156–163. https://doi.org/10.1097/gme.0b013e31817fa9e0

Vaze, N., & Joshi, S. (2010). Yoga and menopausal transition. *Journal of Mid-Life Health*, *1*(2), 56. https://doi.org/10.4103/0976-7800.76212

Vigneswaran, K., & Hamoda, H. (2021). Hormone replacement therapy - current recommendations. *Best Practice & Research Clinical Obstetrics & Gynaecology*, *81*. https://doi.org/10.1016/j.bpobgyn.2021.12.001

Vinogradova, Y., Coupland, C., & Hippisley-Cox, J. (2020). Use of hormone replacement therapy and risk of breast cancer: Nested case-control studies using theQResearch and CPRD databases. *BMJ*, *371*, m3873 https://doi.org/10.1136/bmj.m3873

Vitamin C. (2021, March 26). National Institutes of Health Office of Dietary Supplements, U.S.

Department of Health & Human Services. https://ods.od.nih.gov/factsheets/VitaminC-HealthProfessional/

Vitamin D. (2022, August 12). National Institutes of Health Office of Dietary Supplements, U.S. Department of Health & Human Services. https://ods.od.nih.gov/factsheets/VitaminD-HealthProfessional/

Vitamin E. (2021, March 26). National Institutes of Health Office of Dietary Supplements, U.S. Department of Health & Human Services. https://ods.od.nih.gov/factsheets/VitaminE-HealthProfessional/

Wang, X., Ouyang, Y., Liu, J., Zhu , M., Zhao, G., Bao, W., & Hu, F. B. (2014). Fruit and vegetable consumption and mortality from all causes, cardiovascular disease, and cancer: Systematic review and dose-response meta-analysis of prospective cohort studies. *BMJ, 349*, g4490–g4490. https://doi.org/10.1136/bmj.g4490

Warren, M. P., & Halpert, S. (2004). Hormone replacement therapy: controversies, pros and cons. *Best Practice & Research Clinical Endocrinology & Metabolism, 18*(3), 317–332. https://doi.org/10.1016/j.beem.2004.02.005

Weber, M. T., Mapstone, M., Staskiewicz, J., & Maki, P. M. (2012). Reconciling subjective memory complaints with objective memory performance in the menopausal transition. *Menopause, 19*(7), 735–741.

https://doi.org/10.1097/gme.0b013e318241fd
22

What Is Menopause? (2021, September 30). National
Institute on Aging.
https://www.nia.nih.gov/health/what-
menopause

Whitcomb, B. W., Whiteman, M. K., Langenberg, P.,
Flaws, J. A., & Romani, W. A. (2007). Physical
activity and risk of hot flashes among women in
midlife. *Journal of Women's Health*, *16*(1), 124–133.
https://doi.org/10.1089/jwh.2006.0046

Whitely, C. (n.d.). *Menopause Exercise: The Top 5 Best
Exercises.* Health & Her.
https://healthandher.com/hot-topics/best-
exercise-menopause/

Wisner, W. (2022, October 17). *Understanding the Impact of
Menopause on Mental Health.* Verywell Mind.
https://www.verywellmind.com/menopause-
and-mental-health-symptoms-and-treatments-
6746966

Wobser, R. W., & Takov, V. (2023, May 1). *Black Cohosh.*
PubMed; StatPearls Publishing.
https://www.ncbi.nlm.nih.gov/books/NBK47
0187/

Women's Health Initiative (WHI). (n.d.). National Heart,
Lung, and Blood Institute.
https://www.nhlbi.nih.gov/science/womens-
health-initiative-whi

Wuttke, W., Jarry, H., Haunschild, J., Stecher, G., Schuh, M., & Seidlova-Wuttke, D. (2014). The non-estrogenic alternative for the treatment of climacteric complaints: Black cohosh (*Cimicifuga* or *Actaea racemosa*). *The Journal of Steroid Biochemistry and Molecular Biology*, *139*, 302–310. https://doi.org/10.1016/j.jsbmb.2013.02.007

Xu, Y., Wang, C., Klabnik, J., & O'Donnell, J. M. (2014). Novel therapeutic targets in depression and anxiety: Antioxidants as a candidate treatment. *Current Neuropharmacology*, *12*(2), 108–119. https://doi.org/10.2174/1570159X1166613112 0231448

Yoga, Kegel Exercises, Pelvic Floor Physical Therapy. (n.d.). The North American Menopause Society. https://www.menopause.org/for-women/sexual-health-menopause-online/effective-treatments-for-sexual-problems/yoga-kegel-exercises-pelvic-floor-physical-therapy

Zhang, Y., Wu, H.-Y., Du, J., Xu, J., Wang, J., Tao, C., Li, L., & Xu, H. (2016). Extracting drug-enzyme relation from literature as evidence for drug drug interaction. *Journal of Biomedical Semantics*, *7*, 11. https://doi.org/10.1186/s13326-016-0052-6

Zinman, R. (2020, March 29). *5 Gentle Yoga Poses for Menopause*. Healthline. https://www.healthline.com/health/yoga-for-menopause

Printed in Great Britain
by Amazon

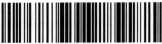

30650641R00090